MOTHER HOOD YOUR WAY

Hollie de Cruz

MOTHER HOOD YOUR WAY

HOW TO WORRY LESS AND ENJOY MORE IN YOUR BABY'S FIRST YEAR

Vermilion

1

Vermilion, an imprint of Ebury Publishing,
20 Vauxhall Bridge Road,
London SW1V 2SA

Vermilion is part of the Penguin Random House group of companies whose addresses can be found at global.penguinrandomhouse.com

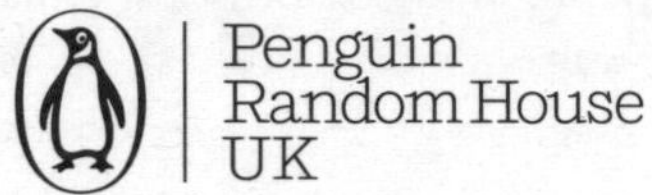

First published by Vermilion in 2021

www.penguin.co.uk

A CIP catalogue record for this book is available from the British Library

ISBN 9781785043147

Printed and bound in Great Britain by Clays Ltd, Elcograf S.p.A.

The authorised representative in the EEA is Penguin Random House Ireland, Morrison Chambers, 32 Nassau Street, Dublin D02 YH68.

To my late, beloved grandfather, Gandy – for your quiet and ongoing commitment to nonconformism. I miss it, and I miss you.

To my incredible children – Oscar and Cosmo, for carrying that magic in your own hearts, and for expanding mine more than you'll ever know.

CONTENTS

INTRODUCTION

On the day my first son was born, the mother in me was, too. I was twenty-five years old, yet I felt as brand new as the little baby in my arms. I felt as vulnerable, as open, and as sensitive, and I wanted to be held, just as he did. Society forgets this. Society forgets that when you give birth, you too are born. I remember feeling like my protective outer shell had been stripped back, and I was left exposed to the elements of newfound motherhood, with a heady cocktail of fear and courage mixed together running through my veins. I'll never forget leaving hospital with my baby a couple of days later. We'd packed up our stuff, wrapped Oscar up for the snowy world that waited outside, and shuffled up to the maternity reception to, I guess, *check out*. 'It's okay, you can just go,' a midwife said. 'Really?' I asked, confused at the apparent nonchalance under which I was permitted to leave with such precious cargo. 'Yes,' she said, 'good luck.'

Good luck.

When we got back to our little flat – our baby now safely tucked up in his car seat instead of my belly – I clearly remember his dad putting him down on the floor of our living room and then looking at me to share a 'do we laugh or do we cry?' moment. This was it. The birth we'd long prepared and practised for was over, and the real work was about to begin. The work we'd never done before. The work we had no how-to guide for. The work we would surely get wrong, and try again at. We were parents. I was a mother, and I had no idea what I was doing.

Thinking back to the first few weeks and months of Oscar's life is now a blur. I was in survival mode. I felt so open, emotionally and physically. My body, which I barely recognised with its engorged boobs, was recovering from a long labour and abdominal birth, while my head and heart were coming to terms with the overwhelming love, fear and responsibility I felt to keep this tiny person safe. I had no idea where to start in terms of processing what I was feeling, and the desire to find some source of control was visceral.

During those night sweats and early-hour feeds, I remember frantically tapping every question under the sun into Google. Why is my baby making strange noises? Is my baby hungry? How do I know if my baby is getting enough milk? Cure for cracked nipples. Silent reflux. What is an osteopath? How to make your baby sleep. What colour should breastmilk be? You name it, I googled it. The whole thing felt a bit like trying to put together a piece of flatpack furniture with twelve different sets of contradictory instructions, and the question I kept asking over and over was 'but how do I know if I'm getting it right?'.

I feel like that question was on repeat in my head for at least the first year of my little one's life. Is he warm enough? Should I persevere with breastfeeding? Do I need to implement a routine? Are we bonding? Should I go back to work? Am I still me? Will I ever go out again? Does everyone think I'm rubbish at this? And repeat x 100. I questioned every move I made, constantly compared myself to everyone else and frequently battled this idea that I wasn't enough. I wasn't maternal enough, loving enough, clever enough, strict enough, organised enough or good enough to be this wonderful boy's mother.

A few years in, and by this point I was now a hypnobirthing teacher. A friend and colleague of mine was telling me about a postnatal ritual called Closing the Bones. A ceremony originating from Ecuador, Closing the Bones is the sacred act of supporting a woman's recovery after her baby's birth. The ritual involves a tight binding – thought to bring a new mother's body back together and prevent her from leaking precious energy, while giving her an offering of stillness to celebrate her amazing achievements. In a space where all is quiet and she is held – a rarity for mothers – she is invited to thank her body for its service, reflect on her emotional journey into motherhood and invite back the part of her soul that left her to make way for that of her baby. I was intrigued and in awe that something would exist to honour the physical and emotional work of the mother in such a beautiful, nurturing way, and I knew I needed to try it for myself. It exceeded all of my expectations and I found myself, while held tightly in the embrace of these binds, feeling deeply emotional, incredibly centred and like I could finally accept and step into who I had become.

After this experience, I began – slowly but surely – to settle into this new part of myself. It was the catalyst I needed to own my experience of motherhood and to have the courage to explore, make mistakes and live in a way that felt right for me. I made space to regularly quieten my thoughts, to turn down the noise of other people's opinions and to exercise the muscles that told me which feelings were mine and which had been planted by the expectations of my society. I went to therapy. I identified some of the influences that had planted these seeds of self-doubt, and unpicked the cycles of behaviour that I knew I didn't want to be part of any more, or didn't want to transfer to my child. It was hard, it was cathartic and it was hugely transformative for me. It led me to explore more about attachment theory, about how our society, media and culture affect the way we parent, and how much the roles of mothers and respect towards them varies around the world.

Ultimately, these experiences are what led me to write this book, partly as a mother but primarily as someone who cares deeply about the experience of women and mothers. On considering motherhood from a universal perspective – rather than the version limited by the expectations put upon us – I could appreciate how personal each journey is. I wanted to explore that, in the hope it would speak to and support the mothers feeling alone or lost along the way. What works for one will trip up another, and there are so rarely solutions that work across the board. Every baby is different and so is every mother, and the joy comes when we embrace our uniqueness and celebrate the call of our own maternal wisdom.

'But what if I don't have a sense of maternal wisdom?' I hear you wonder. Believe me, you do; it may just be tucked away somewhere. It was for me. It was hidden under layers of other people's ideas, my own childhood experiences, the complexities of guilt and a shift in my identity, warped visions of what 'getting it right' looked like, and a fog of fear around the consequence of 'getting it wrong'. It was dictated by whether or not I breastfed, whether my baby slept through the night, whether I made my own purées and whether they would tolerate tummy-time.

When you take away other people's thoughts and beliefs on things like this, you can become more aligned with your own feelings towards them, and that is the start of this process: turning down the outside noise and learning to listen. And that's where we reach the core of our maternal wisdom: our intuition. Eight years after becoming a mother for the first time, I had another baby and I'd be lying if I said those feelings of doubt didn't creep back in. Will I remember what I'm doing? Will this baby be the same? Will breastfeeding be easier? Will he sleep? These thoughts consumed me for a good portion of my pregnancy. I had planned a home birth as I had with my first, but Cosmo – just like his big brother – had other ideas, and decided to enter the world very quickly with another emergency C-section. In the days following his birth, I couldn't get my head around not getting the birth I'd planned (despite all of my hypnobirthing practice!) and then it hit me – go with the flow, expect the unexpected – his birth was a blessing in disguise, and exactly the lesson I needed to realign with my intentions of enjoying things *our way* this time.

And that's exactly what I did. From the day Cosmo was born, I made a conscious effort to be led only by *my* instincts and *his* needs. I have learned to take control of what I can and let go of what I can't; I have learned to say no when I need to, and to put the needs of my children (which in turn, at times, means my own) ahead of anyone else's; and I have learned to be led by my heart rather than the expectations of others. There has been more unlearning and unpacking, more sitting with feelings of discomfort, and more stepping outside of society's comfort zone and back into mine. It has brought with it deeper, richer experiences, a much stronger sense of respect and love for myself, and an avenue to feel joy even in the hardest, darkest, most trying moments. Is it always easy? No. Is it always possible? Yes. It just takes practice. Think of it as exercising your maternal muscles, and if that fills you with fear or unease, don't worry; I'm here to show you how and to support your 'exercise' with practical tips and simple, effective activities. I am writing this book because I believe that learning to enjoy motherhood your way will bring you clarity and confidence on your new adventure, that it will instil a stronger sense of value in the work you're doing, and that it will offer you an opportunity to be present and switched on to the highs and lows of a relationship this special. It starts with you, and it's going to be mega, I promise.

Hopefully you'll soon realise that this book is by no means a manual. I'm not here to tell you how to parent or what your experience should look and feel like. There's no denying there'll be breezy days and '*oh-*

jeezy' days, but I'm hoping you'll find among the pages that follow the reassurance you need, some tools that might make the trickier days that bit easier and, ultimately, the respect and kudos you completely deserve. I have divided the book up into bite-sized segments to cover your baby's first year: The First 48 Hours; The Fourth Trimester; Resurfacing (3–6 months); and Onwards and Upwards (6 months and beyond). Throughout these sections, you'll find some ideas around what to expect, ways to nurture your baby and yourself through the physical and emotional landscape, and how to integrate this journey with those around you, so that you are leaning on and living alongside your support network, rather than expending too much energy trying to please or fit in with them. There are lots of tips for turning down outside parental noise (however well-meaning!), techniques for recalibrating when everything is getting on top of you, and lots of exercises for finding an abundance of joy and embracing Motherhood, Your Way. While I do talk lots about your baby's first year, I think you'll be pleased to discover that the confidence I hope to impart to you takes you way beyond and well into your ongoing growth as a mother. Much as with birth, the tools we learn to remain calm and work with our natural rhythms, rather than against them, naturally filter into everything you do from there, so be open to how these thought processes and practices can create slow and sustainable shifts over the years to come.

I would really encourage you to use this book in a way that feels right for you. You may come across things that don't align with you or that you hadn't considered, and that's okay. And with a topic as broad and diverse as motherhood, it would be impossible for me to cover every nook and cranny, but hopefully you will find lots of insightful, relatable and thought-provoking ideas. Even if something doesn't feel immediately palatable, try sitting with your preconditioned thoughts and work out if there's space for, or even a little magic in, doing things differently. We can often cling on to our learned and lived-in experiences without much thought for things we might like to change, and creating the space to reflect and reprioritise this work can be a hugely rewarding rung on the motherhood ladder.

As a little bonus, and as an extra dose of solidarity and support, you'll have access to my Motherhood Meditation MP3, which has been created as an opportunity for some time out and recalibration. On the days when it's all getting too much and you feel like you don't know what you're doing, take ten minutes out with this MP3 and you'll soon be reminded that you do. The MP3 can be accessed at www.penguin.co.uk/motherhoodyourway.

Remember, too, that one person's experience or opinion is not a criticism of yours. We all do things in our own unique ways, informed by our own beliefs and values, and there is a true beauty in the complex and scenic landscape of motherhood (and childhood) that this creates. Don't be afraid to get things wrong. Get comfortable with changing direction when presented with new resources, and embrace the ultimate journey of getting to know the deepest parts of yourself. At the end of each section, there's space for you to reflect on these ideas and what you've read. Do that in your own way: draw, write, doodle, journal – use the space however you want to, and treasure it as part of your ongoing journey.

You'll also find plenty of positive affirmations throughout the book – consider them your personal cheerleaders over the coming months.

Above all, remember that you are fully equipped, in your heart, to be the exact mother your child needs. You will learn and grow every day, and your baby will teach you more than any book ever will. Think of me as your companion. I'll cheer, you lead.

PART ONE

THE FIRST 48 HOURS

When we're pregnant, we spend a lot of time thinking about and planning for two specific things. The first is our baby's birth. What do I want it to be like? Who is going to support me? Where is it going to happen? Maybe you've taken a hypnobirthing course or attended another type of antenatal education, packed and unpacked your hospital bag multiple times, and spent time researching and rewriting your birth plan. I expect you've created a birth playlist, thought about snacks and practised your breathing techniques ahead of the birth, so that you feel calmer and more confident ahead of your baby's birth day.

The next bit of pre-planning tends to involve what life will look like once your baby's here. Maybe you've bought some clothes, decorated the nursery, researched car seats and test-driven buggies. You will have thought about names, maybe considered childcare options for further down the line, or made changes to your practical set-up at home to make way for this new little person. There are so many adventures ahead and it's exciting to sit and ponder what that's going to look like.

There's no denying that these both deserve thought and planning. They feel so tangible and exciting, and of course they are the elements of parenthood that everyone around you is likely to be talking about, too. In my experience though, it means the immediate period after your baby is born can often get overlooked, when in fact those early days with your newborn are likely to have a huge impact on your onward journey. With this in mind, I want to spend some time helping you to visualise and emotionally prepare for the 48 hours after your baby is born. I want to explore with you what you might be feeling during this time, reassure you that you're doing a great job, and share with you a handful of very simple and effective ideas to help make this short and sacred bubble as enjoyable, relaxing and precious as possible.

Whether you have had a home birth or are recovering in hospital, those first 48 hours with your new baby are likely to be some of the most magical, surprising, overwhelming hours of your life.

> It's okay to feel a bit bewildered or blindsided – you've just done something physically incredible.

And remember that this is a totally new experience for you, your partner (if you have one) and your brand-new baby, whether this is your first baby or your fourth. Take your time and be patient and accepting of each other as you acclimatise and adjust to what life looks like now. Enjoy this special time in a way that feels right for you, and don't expect too much. In these precious hours, your baby needs nothing more than you, and everything you're doing is exactly right.

I know how overwhelming, exciting and exhausting those first 48 hours with your new baby can feel, so before we go any further, I want to give you a super-simple and effective resetting technique that will help calm your system and settle you in the moment, however it is unfolding. This technique requires little thought or practice, so it's a brilliant one to try when your head and heart are full of so many other things. It's a lovely one for when you're holding your baby, and will help you remain open to soaking up these precious moments of getting to know your little one.

I am a strong,
capable woman

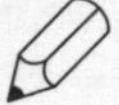

ACTIVITY

HEART SPACE CENTRING

Heart space centring is one of my favourite breathing exercises as it offers a very quick opportunity to mentally relax and release physical tension. It quickly short-circuits our stressor hormones and brings about a welcome sense of peace and ease, grounding us in precious moments. Heart space centring is focused around bringing awareness to our breath, but I don't want you to worry too much about a specific technique at the moment, because you'll learn more about that with the Calm Breath at the end of this section (see page 33).

Simply begin to notice the rise and fall of your breath in this moment. Notice how your heart space grows and then relaxes. Imagine your heart filling with love and light with each breath in, and then, as you breathe out, easily releasing any doubt, thought or feeling that isn't serving you.

As you breathe in (either through your nose or mouth, it doesn't matter right now), say in your mind 'I am safe', and as you breathe out, say in your mind 'all is well'. Breathe these words in and out of your heart and I bet that within three breaths you'll be feeling calmer and more centred.

THE FUNDAMENTAL FOUR

I want to keep things clear, calm and concise for you while we focus on this 48-hour period, so we're going to focus on *The Fundamental Four*. That's you, your baby, your network and your nest.

THE FIRST 48 HOURS AND... YOU

Now, seeing as you're the one who's just brought your beautiful baby into the world, it seems only fair to start with YOU.

> You're a mum. Maybe you were already a mum, maybe you hadn't expected to be a mum or maybe it's been a long time coming. However you've got here: wow. You've done it and for that alone, you are absolutely amazing.

In fact, anchor that in your mind now. If you're reading this ahead of your baby's birth, then I want the first thing you say to yourself when you bring your baby into the world to be, 'I'm amazing, I'm here and I did it.' You can practise it now, and if your baby has already arrived, do the same! 'I'm amazing, I'm here and I did it.'

Whether your baby was born vaginally or abdominally, whether that journey was straightforward or more complicated, it is likely that you're going to be in some kind of physical discomfort in the immediate period following their birth. It is completely normal to

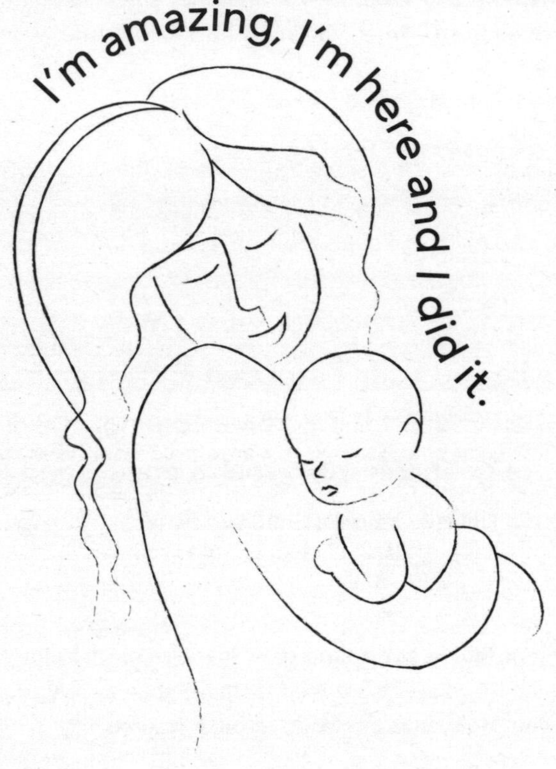
I'm amazing, I'm here and I did it.

experience things like bleeding, after-pains, constipation, swelling, and maybe some soreness if you've had an episiotomy, tearing or stitches. Because we all focus on the physicality of birth itself, these things can often be overlooked in your preparations, so I want to touch on them here to reassure you that they are very common and easily recovered from – when you know how to look after yourself and prioritise them.

Physiological post-birth healing

Bleeding

Whether you've given birth vaginally or abdominally, you will bleed from your vagina afterwards. This blood is called 'lochia' and also includes mucus and uterine tissue, meaning it can appear heavier and brighter than the bleeding you'd experience during a period. This bloody discharge can continue for up to six weeks after your baby's birth, becoming gradually lighter. This is completely normal and it's your body's way of shedding your womb tissue and then replacing the lining after you've given birth. It's very normal to notice clots in this blood, too. However, if they are larger than a 50-pence piece, or you notice a bad smell, then do tell your midwife.

Be sure you have a good quantity of maternity pads (they are much more absorbent than regular sanitary towels) and lots of fresh knickers (go for black!). That way you can remain on top of your bleeding and stay fresh and comfortable after your baby's birth.

After-pains

Strangely, even when your baby has been born, it can feel like you're still experiencing contractions or tightenings in your uterus, a sensation that can increase when you breastfeed. It is simply your uterine muscle contracting back to its smaller size now that there's no baby to accommodate. These sensations tend to be stronger in women who have already had a baby, but some women don't experience them very noticeably at all. Remember that every woman's body works in its own way. If you're experiencing a lot of discomfort with this, you can ask your midwife for some pain relief, or use a warm compress over your back, tummy (check with your midwife first if you've had an abdominal birth), or wherever the pain is presenting. It's also a great idea to use the Calm Breath on page 33 to soften your body, relax your muscles and help lessen the discomfort of these sensations.

Trapped wind or constipation

Your body has worked so hard during labour and birth that it can sometimes take a few days for your digestive system to re-regulate and settle back into its normal rhythm. The best way to encourage this is to make sure you are drinking plenty of water and grazing on foods that are fibrous. Things like prunes, figs, pears and apples make for easy fibrous snacks (up your water intake accordingly so as not to make matters worse!). Think about including some of these in your birth bag for the days after your baby's birth, whether that's at home or in hospital. Your bowels should open naturally within two or three days, but it's really important that you remain relaxed and avoid straining when passing your first bowel movement. Use the Calm Breath again, or channel the control and focus you used to bring your baby into the world! Soften, breathe, relax. Your body knows what it's doing, so follow its lead.

Constipation can often lead to the pain associated with trapped wind, and this is often more common after an abdominal birth. If you can address the constipation, this pain should subside naturally, but if it's too uncomfortable you can ask your midwife for some laxatives or an enema to bring about relief more quickly. It's also worth bearing in mind that for a small percentage of people, constipation may be caused by other underlying issues and could be made worse by eating more fibre. If you feel like this is you, do speak to your care providers. Never feel embarrassed about addressing your concerns with your midwives – they are there to support and comfort you, and they are used to helping women with these issues day in, day out.

Tearing/stitches

If you've had stitches after tearing or an episiotomy, or have a small tear that is being left to heal naturally, the area can feel sore in the days following your baby's birth. It's important to keep the area clean and dry: bathe in plain warm water and then pat yourself dry gently with a clean towel. Lying on your side or propping yourself up against the softness of cushions can really help you feel more comfortable, and again, you can ask your midwife for painkillers if you would like them. There is certainly no shame in asking for pain relief; it will free you up to focus on your baby and enjoy these first days. Remember that no one is judging you, and everyone wants to help.

I am kind to and go gently with my hard-working body

Looking after yourself is a way of looking after your baby, too. So don't keep quiet if you're worried about something. It's equally normal to experience all, none or some of these post-birth symptoms. In the immediate period following your baby's birth, you'll have midwives on hand to help and support you, so it makes sense to use this to your advantage and ask them about anything you're unsure of, however silly or insignificant it may seem.

Physical symptoms that may be a sign of something more serious can include a severe headache or blurred vision, swelling in your legs, clots that are larger than a 50-pence piece or a high fever. Talk to your midwife immediately if you notice any of these changes; they can give you the help you need quickly.

The emotional landscape of the first two days

All the emotions

While the physical post-birth happenings might feel all-consuming, let's not forget how much is going on hormonally and emotionally, too. On a rational level (and when we're not in the midst of it!), it makes complete sense that we are overcome with all sorts of feelings in the hours that follow our baby's birth. Don't forget that at the time, you're also dealing with fluctuating hormones and sleep deprivation/exhaustion, especially if you've experienced a long labour. Lots of women describe the immediate postnatal period as 'a blur', and I think this is often because we don't know how to process so much in such a short space of time. I often wonder if this experience of an 'emotional blackout' is a coping mechanism of sorts; and needless to say it can also be influenced by a birth not going to plan, or extra elements to your physical recovery that you weren't expecting.

Another stumbling block in the early days with your newborn is the image in your pre-kids mind versus the *we've-just-had-a-baby* reality. We have these logged subconscious images of families waiting excitedly in the hospital corridor, bursting in with balloons when the first cries are heard, while Mum sits up in bed, doe-eyed and glowy-cheeked, gushing over her new bundle of neatly wrapped joy. There's no denying that the immediate aftermath of meeting your baby is full of excitement and oxytocin, but it's important to allow space for the breadth of emotions it's normal to feel in those first few days. There will be lots of feels to feel, and the more open you are to these being normal, the more likely you are to be able to process them calmly, without spiralling into any kind of panic – and, most brilliantly, able to retain valuable memories of this time.

Normal emotional experiences among the chaos of those early days may include, but are not limited to: excitement, overwhelm, intense love, fear, vulnerability, pride, anxiety, teariness, happiness, sadness, joy, anger, doubt, relief, sensitivity, exhaustion, invincibility.

That's a big load of feelings, right? When we feel overloaded with feelings – especially ones that we'd usually consider to clash – we can end up feeling almost a sense of 'nothing'. These feelings get blurred and lost and it can sometimes lead to a lot of anxiety or emotional discomfort around our experience.

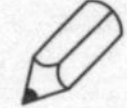

ACTIVITY

BABY BUBBLE BALLOONS

I want to give you the opportunity here to recognise all the feelings you are experiencing while you're in this precious bubble of time. This really simple but effective activity will not only help you to process what you are feeling as and when you're ready to, but will also help to ground you in the present moment and retain positive, meaningful memories to take forward and of course look back on.

On the opposite page, you'll see lots of balloons, each containing a different feeling or emotion. When people ask 'how are you feeling?' it's almost too big a question and we often default to 'fine'. Sometimes we need a helping hand in spotting our feelings, especially when we're exhausted, and that's exactly what this easy exercise is going to help facilitate.

What I want you to do is to colour in any balloon that holds an emotion you can relate to or have felt in this 48-hour period. You could use the same colour or mix it up, and there are some balloons that have been left blank for you to add to if you feel like it. Colouring in each balloon acts as an acknowledgement of that feeling, and will help you to reflect and process it

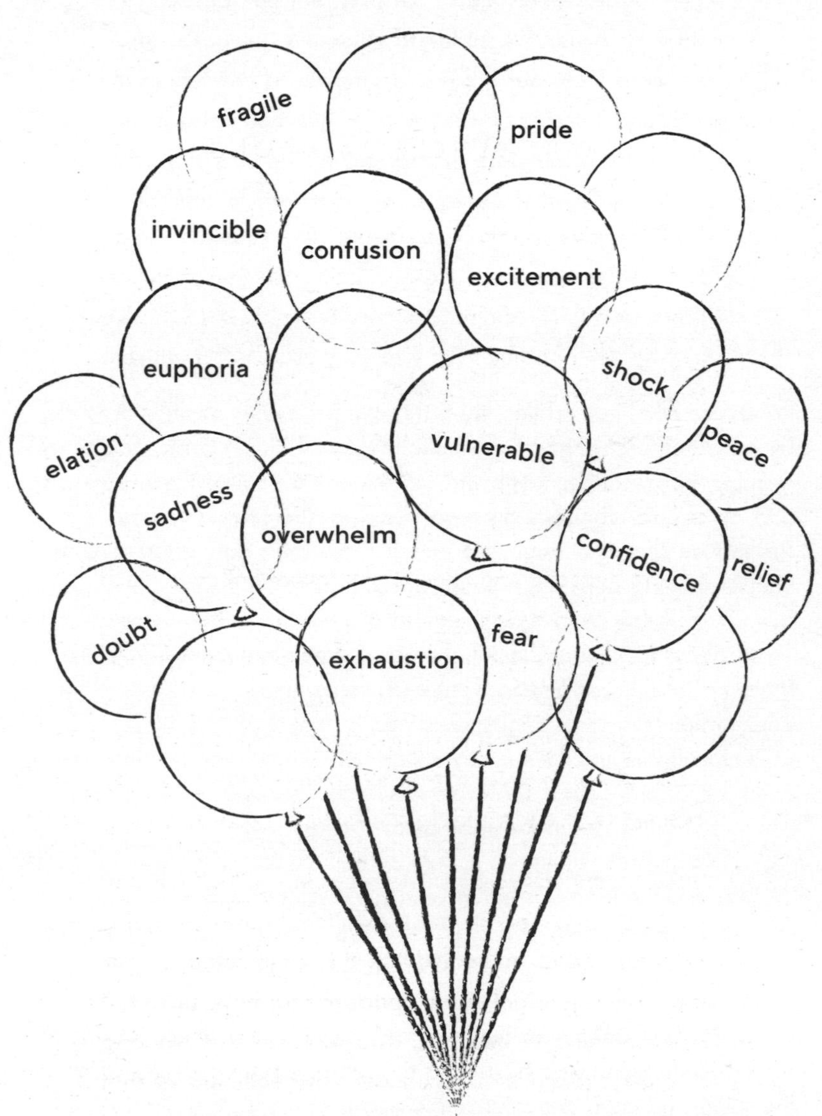
fragile
pride
invincible
confusion
excitement
euphoria
shock
elation
vulnerable
peace
sadness
overwhelm
confidence
relief
doubt
exhaustion
fear

when the time feels right. Not only that but, amazingly, colouring-in has the ability to relax the amygdala (the 'fear centre') in our brains. In working to quieten your mind and focus your attention, it has been shown to induce the same state as meditating. Inviting in these elements of mindfulness will allow your brain to 'breathe'.

THE FIRST 48 HOURS AND... YOUR BABY

When our baby first arrives, we are blown away (for obvious reasons) by how much changes for us. So many of our 'norms' suddenly change, our priorities shift, and we experience all of these physical and emotional changes that we have to slowly get to grips with. Among all of this change, it's easy to overlook how enormous the effects of being born are on your baby, too.

Think about it. In a matter of moments they have transitioned from this dark, small, warm space where all of their needs are met instantly and completely, to a bright, loud world where they have to shout for help all the time! It's a really big deal, and I think it often gets overlooked in a culture that obsesses about routine, order, being in control, and the idea of how things are *meant* to be.

We are sold the idea of what babies are meant to look like, how they are meant to behave, and even how we should ideally cope with/ manage their new life with us. A 'good' baby is one who sleeps well and doesn't cry much, right? Now read that back to yourself. This is a new baby. A baby who depends on you for every single branch of their existence and who hasn't got the memo about the rules of what the society it's born into deems important.

With that in mind, I want to take the opportunity to dispel a few myths around newborn behaviour and help you to find ways to nurture your baby through their transition Earthside, without losing your marbles.

Sleep, eat, repeat

In the early days and weeks of your baby's life, it is completely normal for them to sleep more in the day than they do at night. It is very, very unlikely that your baby will have, need or benefit from any kind of routine around sleep at this stage, because there is so much that is changing in a very short space of time and their sleep needs adapt in order to help them adjust to and process these changes.

When your baby is born, their stomach is roughly the size of a cherry, which means it fills and empties really quickly. When you can get your head around this (and see the illustration on page 104), I find it really helps to understand why they want/need to feed so frequently and sleep in regular, seemingly short blocks. For this reason, it is incredibly unlikely that your baby will sleep through the night (six to eight hours) before the age of three months, but also very normal for them not to do this before the age of twelve to eighteen months. More about that on page 98.

On the subject of feeding, it's also important to understand the role of colostrum here. Colostrum, fondly known as 'nature's first food', is the thick, golden-coloured milk that you will be producing in the days after your baby's birth. It's very concentrated (hence the darker colour), meaning your baby only needs a tiny amount at a time, while they get used to their new way of eating. In these first 48 hours, it's very normal for your baby to feed every hour or so. When your milk comes in around day three, these feeds become gradually fewer and longer. If you are choosing to breastfeed, then encouraging your baby to suck will stimulate your supply and help encourage good milk production.

Even if you know you are not going to breastfeed on your onward journey, giving your baby just a few feeds of colostrum has unparalleled health benefits, including (but not limited to) strengthening your baby's immunity and supporting the healthy development of their gut.

Closeness and skin-to-skin contact with your baby during these first 48 hours is hugely supportive to their developing sleeping and eating skills. Your baby's sleep is also affected by how safe and comfortable they feel. You may notice that your baby only wants to sleep on you or your partner. Even when you think they are sound asleep, you try to put them down and gah – they're awake! Again, try to put yourself in your baby's booties here. They've been tightly bundled up in a dark, warm place for months, with the sound of your insides and heartbeat for comfort – it's little wonder that this continues to offer them the reassurance they require to rest now that they're in the big wide world. You are their ONLY constant, and you can think of it as your job to help teach them that the world is safe, and make their transition a more gentle and secure one.

Holding your baby, letting them sleep on you, or rocking them is not a bad thing. You are not going to 'make a rod for your own back' or 'create bad habits' or anything else you might have been told by your mum's next-door neighbour's cousin.

There are going to be some exercises as you work through this book that will help you identify and nurture a healthy attachment relationship with your baby, but in these first few days and weeks, all you need to be confident in is that you CANNOT spoil your baby. Promise.

Bonding with your baby

There are no hard and fast rules about how you should bond with your baby, and while lots of us worry about how readily it will happen, we're better off focusing on looking after ourselves emotionally and physically so that we can be available to our baby and let bonding happen more naturally. When we are relaxed and at ease, we become more attuned to our own calls of love and connection, and this is the language you and your baby will communicate in over the coming months. Let's think about what bonding might look like in these very early days, and how you (and your partner if you have one) can open up these wonderful channels through which love and connectedness can flow.

Skin-to-skin

In the first few days after birth (and of course beyond), you can both enjoy skin-to-skin cuddles with your baby. It is easy, costs nothing and is one of the most simple and powerful ways to bond with your baby. Skin-to-skin contact not only helps to regulate baby's body temperature and heart rate in the hours and days that follow their birth, but it also helps to comfort and reassure them through sound and smell, and allows you to soak up that gorgeous newborn scent that instigates the production of all of our love and attachment hormones. Going forward, and if your whereabouts won't always allow for skin-to-skin, then baby-wearing can be a brilliant alternative. Carrying your baby in a sling means they benefit from being close to your skin, smell and heartbeat, while you have your hands free! Jersey wrap slings are a brilliant option in the newborn days, as the soft but secure hold replicates being in the womb and as such is super-comforting.

Talk to baby

Remember that even though your baby has only just arrived, they've been listening to you and your partner's voices for a long time. Babies are extremely receptive and responsive to familiar sounds in the womb (it's why they love white noise so much!), so those voices they've heard most often during your pregnancy are likely to be calming for your little one now, too. Now you may feel strange talking to a baby who has no idea what you're saying, but the joy is, they really don't care. Tell your baby what you're doing or how you feel. Tell them about their family, your friends, your wishes for them or how you decided on their name. Getting to talk unapologetically like this to a captive audience can be surprisingly therapeutic!

Enjoying a story or a song

Reading a story or singing a song can be a wonderful way to bond with your baby, and also helps to build familiarity through the comfort of repetition. There was a song that I remember my grandmother singing to me when I was really tiny (it's actually one of my earliest memories). It was called 'Golden Slumbers' and after I had my second son, I found that Elbow had recorded a version of it, which then became my special song with him – one I've gone on to sing at bedtime or when he needs settling, reassurance or comfort. Is there a song or a story that you or your partner remember from childhood? Feelings of nostalgia and happy memories naturally trigger the production of endorphins, which makes for an even more optimal environment in which bonding can happen, and this applies to all of you.

Mirror your baby's movements

We're going to talk about this more in the next section (see page 129), but this is a really simple way to interact with your baby even in these very early days, and opens up the first channels for communication while deepening the bond between you. Holding your baby or lying down by their side, copy their movements and facial expressions. While you may not get any reactions for a while yet, don't underestimate how much your baby is taking in and the closeness it's creating between you.

I am exactly what my baby needs

THE FIRST 48 HOURS AND… YOUR SUPPORT NETWORK

Needless to say, your focus in these first 48 hours is going to be on the brand-new human in your arms. Not only will you be feeding them and sustaining them completely, but you will also be switching on all of these new instincts and senses that enable you to take care of your baby. Remember though that at this time you are also in the midst of your physical and emotional recovery, and that means that YOU need looking after, too. I always like to think of it, as with labour, of Mum looking after her little one while her loved ones look after her. Now this doesn't necessarily need to be your partner; we could be talking about a mother, sister, friend or doula as your support network here. You're also still likely to be under the close care of your midwives and/or obstetrician, so take comfort and reassurance from these people who are here to hold and support you.

In the first 48 hours, your midwives will be helping support your post-partum recovery – checking stitches or a C-section wound, helping you to have a shower and go to the toilet, giving you support to establish breast- or bottle-feeding, and checking that you are feeling physically well. It's really important that you exercise the 'asking for help' muscle, as it's often something that doesn't come too easily. If you feel like something isn't quite right, or want your mind set at ease or a question answering, please, please, please ask your midwives while they are right on hand. It's their job (and passion) to support women in this way, and leaning on their wisdom will help to strengthen yours.

Your birth partner (whether this is your partner or another person) should remain an advocate for you in the hours following your baby's birth. The more you can involve them in your pregnancy and birth, the more confident they will feel in carrying this role forward, and you will be the one ultimately benefitting from this kind of advocacy and support. Obviously, every relationship is different, and we all find our own dynamics in terms of supporting each other. The way they will support you in these first two days will vary, but could include:

Keeping you fed and watered

When you're so focused on meeting the needs of your little one, it can be easy to forget your own, so it's great if your partner, a family member or your extended support network can take on that role in this pocket of time. They can make sure you're keeping really well hydrated and bring you nutritious and fibrous snacks, which might also help to combat the constipation we talked about earlier.

Making sure you're comfortable

If you're in hospital, it's no secret that the beds aren't the comfiest, so your partner can help boost your comfort levels in simple ways. This could mean plumping up your pillows each time you get up so that it's more comfortable when you sit back down, or making sure you have something soft and padded to sit on if you've had stitches or have post-birth haemorrhoids. There's also a wonderful technique called Soothing Strokes, which helps the body to produce endorphins and oxytocin very quickly. While it's a technique that you may have used in your birth, it's an equally useful tool to use in the hours following it, and a lovely one for your partner to do on you while you feed or rest, to restore a sense of calm. We'll talk about this more later on, but for now, the technique can be found on page 117.

Maintaining a calm environment

In a moment we're going to be exploring ways to make a temporary nest in these first two days, but there's lots your partner can do here to help create a calming space. It could be as simple as keeping lights dim, playing some calming music into headphones for you, or popping a few drops of your favourite essential oil onto a cloth for you to inhale.

In terms of your wider support network, you may have invited them to visit you soon after your birth or you may have decided to wait until you are more settled at home. Either way, make sure you are doing what feels right for YOU, and not acting in the interests of other people, or through obligation. This is the one time in your life when you really do get to be unapologetically 'selfish' (although I hate that word!) and completely prioritise yourself and your baby. You may feel like showing off your baby to your closest companions as soon as possible, in which case I'd suggest keeping visits short and sweet so that it doesn't encroach on your valuable rest or feeding. Make some clear decisions on this yourself, or ask your partner or a close family member to take control of the boundaries here and make sure everyone is on the same (your) page. Alternatively, you may feel like preserving this tiny pocket of time as an opportunity for you and your baby (and your partner if you have one) to get to know each other in an undisturbed way. There will be plenty of time to introduce your baby to your loved ones over the coming weeks, so putting yourselves first like this is really no bad thing, and could even prove beneficial to your healing and recovery.

Other ways to utilise your support network in the days following your baby's birth could include:

- Asking them to prepare a meal for the coming days
- Help at home (perhaps putting a wash on, or picking up any groceries you might need)
- Watering house plants or taking care of animals/other children if you need to stay or go into hospital for any reason
- Seeing if they can pick up your favourite snacks if they're coming to see you
- If you've forgotten any essentials for baby or you, they could pick these up too

If you're not the sort of person who finds it easy to ask for help, try to remember that by accepting help you are making yourself more available for your baby. People helping you is people helping your baby and your new family, and when you hear the phrase 'it takes a village', this is what it's all about. If the idea of asking for practical and emotional support in this way still leaves you feeling uncomfortable, then try to make space for a conversation about it with those closest to you ahead of your baby's birth. If you've had an opportunity to tell them how you feel and how they can best support you before your baby arrives, everything will feel more comfortable and seamless on the other side. Remember that asking for help is a sign of strength and that actually, people like to feel useful and helpful, especially when there's a new baby on the scene. Involving people in a way that makes your transition into parenthood easier and more relaxed will make them feel great, and you too! Honestly – you can do it.

We'll go into a bit more detail about asking for help later in the book, but if you want to skip ahead to that now, you can find it on page 73.

I am not afraid to ask for help and lean on those who love me

THE FIRST 48 HOURS AND... YOUR NEST

Whether you're at home, or in the hospital or birth centre, a calm and quiet space immediately post-birth will not only make you feel more relaxed, it will also be hugely beneficial to your baby as they adjust to their monumental transition into the big wide world. Being mindful of this transition, and trying to ensure that it remains a gentle one, can really help your experience of these two days.

Dimmed lighting, music that makes you feel calm and smells that relax and rejuvenate you will all help to create a prolonged intimate space and be beneficial to both you and your baby. Here are some practical tips you could consider whether you're at home or away:

	Home	Away
Lighting	Dimmed lights, candles, fairy lights	LED candles to create a calming glow If you're on a ward, use an eye mask to sleep
Sound	Continue playing your birth playlist	Play your music through headphones
Smells	Inhale essential oils from a tissue/flannel	Inhale essential oils from a tissue/flannel
Comfort	Get into bed, use pillows and blankets	Take a pillow from home and use blankets for comfort

Now that we have explored the magical mayhem that is the first couple of days (and nights) following your baby's birth, I want to share with you a really simple and effective breathing technique that's going to become your go-to reset tool in moments of stress, and prove especially useful at many moments during the 48-hour period following your baby's birth. It's called the Calm Breath and we use it for just that – in the moments where we need to restore a sense of calm despite what might be going on around us.

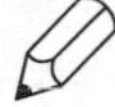

ACTIVITY

THE CALM BREATH

The Calm Breath helps to short-circuit the production of adrenaline – our stressor hormone. It encourages the production of endorphins – our happy hormones – and helps us to feel calmer and more at ease very quickly. You'll certainly find this breath really useful in the days that immediately follow your baby's birth, but it will prove valuable as an accompaniment to your onward journey into parenthood, too. Give it a try:

1. Wherever you are and whatever you're doing, try to place your feet flat on the ground and relax your arms and legs as much as you can. Think of quite literally *grounding* yourself in this moment. Feeling the floor underneath your feet can be really useful for this.
2. Release any tension in your jaw by placing your tongue behind your upper teeth, and allow your shoulders to gently sink down into the frame of your body.
3. You can close your eyes or keep them open, but try to soften the area around them – release any frown or tension in your eyebrows, and soften any worry lines.

We naturally hold a lot of tension behind our eyes, and becoming aware of it can help us to let it go.

4. Take a slow breath in through your nose to a count of four. Visualise the word 'peace', or say 'inhale peace' in your mind as you breathe in.
5. Slowly breathe out through your nose, but try to make this out-breath last for six counts. Visualise the world 'tension', or say 'exhale tension' in your mind as you breathe out.
6. Repeat for 3–5 minutes.

This calming breathing exercise can be done anywhere and at any time, and will become easier and more effective the more you practise it.

Use your Calm Breath as often as you can. Our breath is a bit like a muscle, and the more we exercise it, the stronger it gets. Use it before and during a feed, when you need to pass one of those first bowel movements, whenever your baby cries, if you're suffering with aches and pains when getting up and down, before you go to sleep, and whenever else it could make what you're experiencing that little bit easier and more comfortable.

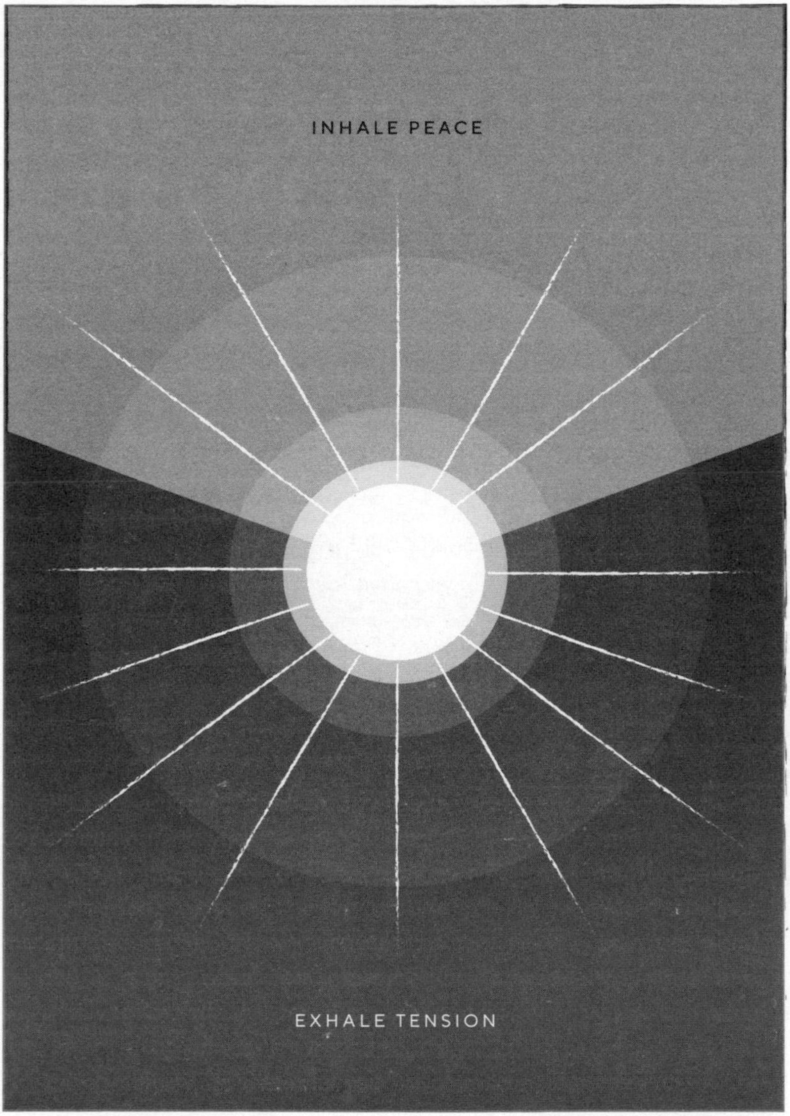

INHALE PEACE

EXHALE TENSION

A FINAL THOUGHT

The thing I want you to really hold on to in these first 48 hours following your baby's birth is how very capable you are.

> However overwhelmed you may feel at times, however out of your depth or exhausted or emotional, you can do this, you really, really can.

Being frightened is a sign that you're doing something really brave, and being scared doesn't mean you're getting it wrong. Yes, your baby has just been born, but you have too. Nurture yourself and offer yourself the sensitivity and gentleness that you are passing down to your baby.

There is no right or wrong, and you are at the start of a slow and rewarding journey of finding *your* way. These are your rules to write, and you can adapt and revise them as much as you like! You and your baby have just arrived here, and these next few weeks are going to be all about getting to know each other and learning together. Be open to what your baby teaches you along the way, as it will help you tune in to that incredible maternal wisdom and love that lies within you. And even if it has not been a habit of your life so far, trust your instincts. They are messages from the mother within, and will always lead you to the answers you can't find anywhere else.

PART TWO

THE FOURTH TRIMESTER

Before we go any further, I want you to take a moment to pat yourself on the back (or wrap your arms around yourself and give yourself a squeeze!) for where you've made it to. Those first 48 hours with your baby can feel full of joy, love and excitement, but they can also feel overwhelming and daunting, especially if you've never done this before! You're probably feeling like you've done little more than *survive* in these early days, but give yourself more credit, Mama – you have kept your little one warm, safe and fed, and you've done more than survived – you've *thrived* (even if it doesn't feel like that yet). Really.

Now that you're slowly starting to recover from your baby's birth, you can begin to immerse yourself in this fourth trimester – a so aptly named part of both your and your baby's journey.

The first three months of your baby's life are best considered an extension of their time inside you and approaching this time as such makes for a much easier transition into what lies ahead.

For nine months, you have been meeting your baby's every need and they have been completely and consistently taken care of inside your womb. Although they make a very physical journey when they are born, their emotional needs remain much the same, and it is our job as mothers to facilitate a continued sense of unconditional love and reassurance for them.

The next few months are going to be precious, but are also likely to feel overwhelming at times. I always think the fourth trimester feels a bit like taking a sabbatical from real life – like you're stepping off the treadmill of societal norms and existing in your own little bubble for a while. It can feel really daunting to take a step away from 'normal life' like this. We might be worried that we'll lose a sense of ourselves, fall out of the loop with our peers or colleagues, and lag behind the fast pace of popular culture and current affairs. It's normal for that to feel scary, but if we look it at from a different perspective, we can begin to consider its sacred nature, and its benefits. Equally, maybe you've been preparing and looking forward to this new adventure for some time, and you find yourself immersed in the moment without a second thought to the pre-baby structures you've stepped out of. There isn't a right or wrong way to feel here – it's really about acknowledging your truth, your experience and embracing the feelings that come up along the way.

No matter what we're up to, life goes on and society continues. Stepping out of that for a little while doesn't mean it's going anywhere, and the experiences you can have during your baby's fourth trimester – if you are willing to immerse yourself in it and embrace it – can be so enriching to your own emotional landscape and onward journey. Our experiences of motherhood can put us in touch with our own energy and resilience, offer perspective on our priorities, and take us to the edges of our physical and emotional strength in a way that, at times, will make us feel invincible. Remember that you don't always need to be travelling in the same direction, or at the same pace, as other people. There is so much joy to be found in being where you are and giving yourself bravely to that time and space. Hopefully you'll start to see that this can be celebrated and that you are not missing out on anything.

The busy world will be there for you to return to when the time is right, but trust that right now, you are exactly where you're meant to be.

With this in mind, I want to give you a really great technique for centring yourself in this belief, especially when your brain might be fighting to tell you otherwise. The Breather Branches technique can be used often on your onward journey, and the more you practise it, the more effective it will become.

ACTIVITY

BREATHER BRANCHES

Breather Branches is a simple technique that will allow you to press pause and re-centre yourself – to give yourself a much-needed breather. It's a really great one to try when you feel like you're falling out of the societal loop or missing out. Often, when we're chasing the past or a more familiar memory of normality, we miss what's happening right in front of us and end up feeling neither here nor there. Using the visualisation of a tree and its branches can really help us take strength in feeling rooted, and help ground us to the time and place we're in (even when it might be unknown or uncomfortable).

Stretching out your hand and thinking of your fingers like the branches of a tree, you're going to trace around them while tuning in to the rhythm of your breath. Look at the illustration opposite, and have a go yourself using these simple steps:

1. Hold out your hand and stretch your fingers so that they resemble the branches of a tree.
2. Using the index finger of your other hand, begin to trace along the hand that you've fanned out.

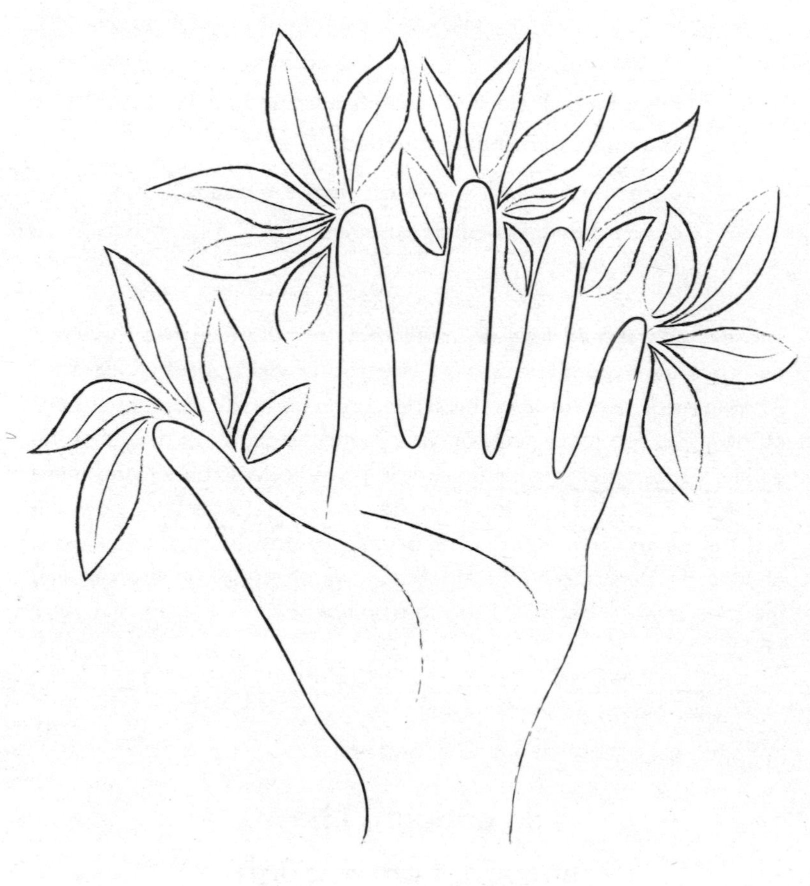

3. As you climb a 'branch', breathe in through your nose and visualise the strength of a tree and all it embodies: strength, growth, nature.
4. As you descend a branch, breathe out through your mouth and visualise the resilience of your tree and the feelings that signifies: withstanding bad weather, letting go, remaining grounded.
5. Continue this until you've reached the opposite side of your hand. Repeat as required.

This exercise should take no more than a minute or two, and can be repeated depending on how stressed or disconnected you feel. As you trace around your breather branches, you can also focus on how this soft touch feels on your hands; becoming aware of the gentle sensation of movement can help you to feel calmer and more relaxed. It's a good idea too to jot down a word to describe how you feel before using your breather branches, and then another word afterwards. Recognising the small positive effects of an exercise like this means you'll be more likely to use it again.

I do enough, I have enough, I am enough

MEETING YOUR BABY'S NEEDS

In our culturally affected and socially influenced adult brains we are quick to assume that what a baby needs is a calm nursery and cosy Moses basket, but a lot of what I'm going to be encouraging you to do in this fourth trimester involves trying to consider things from your baby's perspective, and right now, the only thing they care about is *closeness*. We're going to explore many examples of attachment theory in practice throughout this book, but essentially, your baby doesn't want to be alone, and the secret to a healthy and happy fourth trimester is to acknowledge your invisible work here as being of profound and unsurpassable value.

The main principle of attachment theory centres around emotional and physical availability. A parent who strives to remain responsive to their baby's needs allows that child to develop an innate sense of security as they grow. This means that your baby becomes fully trusting of your dependability, which creates a safe and secure base for them to confidently explore the world around them. Our first attachment relationships are with our primary caregivers, which is why I place so much stress on this invisible work of yours being of such value.

A really great exercise that I often invite new mums (and women in their last trimester of pregnancy) to have a go at is to really visualise what a womb feels like to the baby in it. I know that sounds strange (because how can we possibly know what it's like in there?), but just try to think about it from your baby's perspective. This is a very simple activity that can really help to inform your mindset and approach to the next few months.

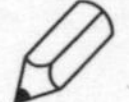

ACTIVITY

MAKING WOMB

Imagine that you are back to being a tiny baby, growing in your mother's womb. You, as yet, have no concept of the outside world that awaits you. You don't know what the rules or expectations are, you don't know what things look like or feel like and you can't do anything for yourself. All you know is the space you currently occupy. Take yourself there, and jot down some words around the questions I've asked below (on the space overleaf). Try not to use your adult knowledge or perspective. Try to keep your thinking simple, primal and through the senses of a baby.

What does it feel like in here?

Is it cold, warm, snug or roomy? Describe what your surroundings feel like.

What does it sound like in here?

Is it quiet or loud? What kind of sounds can I hear?

What does it look like in here?

What can I see? Can I make any shapes or colours out?

What do I need in here?

What do I find reassuring? What do I rely on?

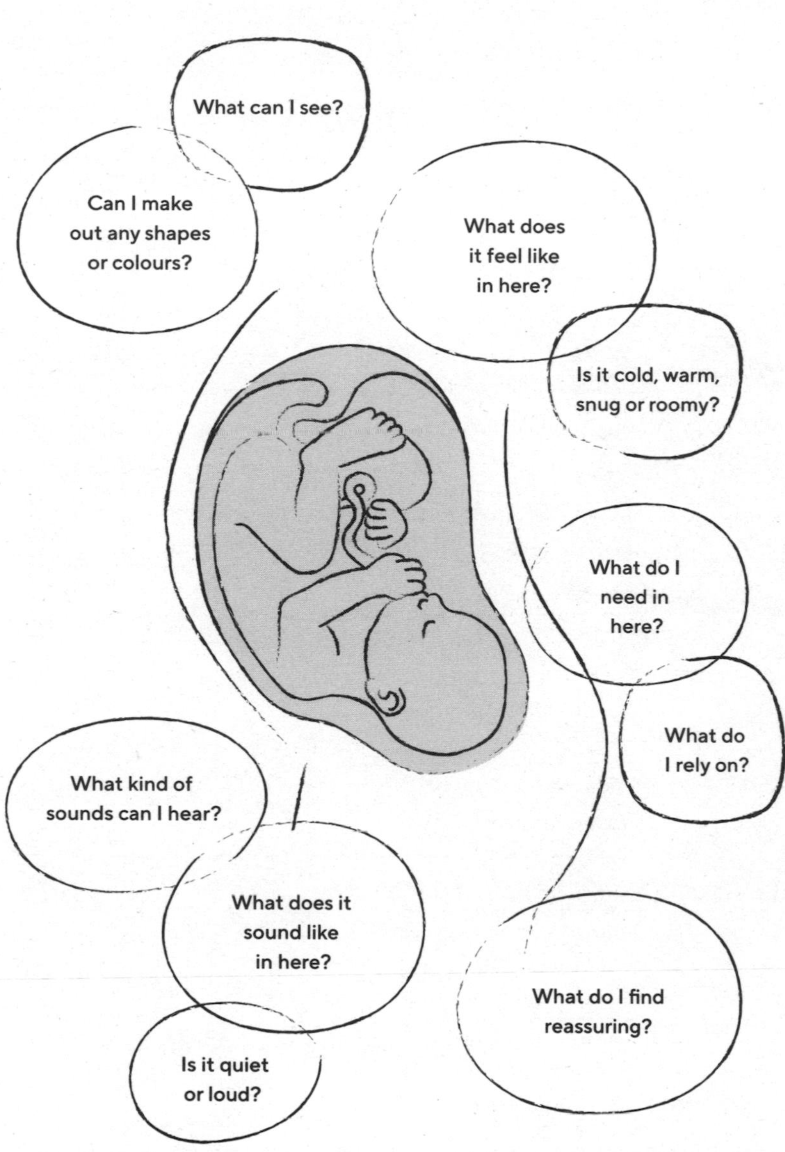
What can I see?
Can I make out any shapes or colours?
What does it feel like in here?
Is it cold, warm, snug or roomy?
What do I need in here?
What do I rely on?
What kind of sounds can I hear?
What does it sound like in here?
Is it quiet or loud?
What do I find reassuring?

When you've completed this exercise, you might notice that your perspective and feelings towards what to expect from your baby begin to shift. Hopefully you'll realise that their needs are incredibly simple. It can be so tempting to overcomplicate what your baby needs and what is required from us, but when we strip things back to what they're used to – warmth, closeness, being fed on demand and familiarity – we become better equipped at embracing the basic (albeit relentless) nature of their requirements.

What often complicates things is our desire to regulate their needs quickly. Try to remind yourself of this over the next few months and consider this fourth trimester a time to recreate the environment they've suddenly emerged from, and ease them into this big, bright new one gently.

When we take a moment to consider things from our baby's perspective, it gives us more insight into what they really need and helps us to slow down and reduce the outside noise of societal expectations – freeing up our minds and hearts to remain exactly where they're needed.

Now, I know what you're thinking. Seeing things through my baby's eyes; doing nothing more than cuddling; and writing off the next few months of being a functioning human being to meet the needs of my baby sounds all well and good in principle, but how? How on earth am I meant to do that when I've just given birth, been catapulted into some slightly sweaty, sleep-poor reality, and am trying to not lose my marbles and cling on to a fading sense of myself? How?

First of all, take a deep breath. Second of all, let me tell you that every single mother, I believe, feels that way. What matters isn't getting it right (there's no such thing), but offering yourself the kindness, compassion and space to go slowly and work it out *your way*, one day at a time. When you start to think of these next three months as an extension of your pregnancy, you'll begin to shift your focus away from outside expectations and towards nurturing your inner experiences, and that's exactly what I'm here to help you do.

I take each day as it comes and follow my baby's lead

MAKING YOUR NEST

In the last chapter, we considered the ways you could bring a sense of calm familiarity to your temporary nest, but now we want to explore how we can make these feelings a bit more permanent. Just as you spent time creating your nest for labour and birth, we should consider the importance of carrying through this sentiment to your postnatal period. At a time when you might be feeling emotionally open and physically more fragile than usual, it is so important that you can relax into your surroundings. Feeling at ease not only encourages you to relax physically, it also means you can lean into the vulnerability of this sacred and transitional time.

Making your nest will also allow you to feel completely relaxed and more available to meet the simple needs of your baby. In the Making Womb exercise, we considered what it is our baby actually needs to make their transition Earthside a more gentle and secure one, and by creating a nest that feels safe and sacred for you both, you'll be better equipped to do this.

So what does it take to create your newborn nest?

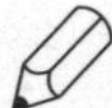

ACTIVITY

THE NEWBORN NEST

Now that you're a few days into life with your baby, or maybe home from hospital if that's where you had your baby, it's a really good idea to make yourself as physically comfortable as possible in your newborn nest. The more physically comfortable you feel, the more you will be able to relax and ease into the more demanding moments of life with your newborn baby. If you had a pregnancy cushion (you know those sausage-shaped ones that you wrapped your restless legs around?), then it can double up brilliantly as a feeding cushion, which can make it much easier to achieve comfortable positioning for you and your baby.

If you've had a winter baby, think about having a cosy blanket, heatable wheat packs (great for sore muscles)

or a hot-water bottle on hand. If you've had a summer baby, think about things like cooling eye masks that you can keep in the fridge, a fan, or a small tub that you can fill with cool water and pop your feet in while you're on the sofa. It's small things like this that can really instil a sense of feeling looked after and nurtured, and that puts you in the best possible position to pass that same care on to your baby.

When we're trying to relax our minds, we want to appeal to all of our physical senses. So think about smells, sounds, sights and so on. Consider what makes you feel happy, calm and at ease when it comes to these physical senses.

Smells

What are your favourite smells? Perhaps there's a candle or essential oil that you loved using during pregnancy – make sure you're stocked up so that you can enjoy it postnatally too. While you should avoid diffusing oils around babies younger than three months old, you could still pop a few drops on a flannel or handkerchief to inhale when you make a cup of tea or get into bed at night. Alternatively, it may be that you can use it in the bath, or by rubbing it into your arms and legs after a shower to rejuvenate and relax yourself. Your baby will find the smell of YOU the most comforting thing of all, so lots of skin-to-skin and physical closeness will be hugely reassuring to them in these early weeks. Wearing your baby in a soft jersey wrap sling can be convenient when you're moving around, and comforting for them, so everyone wins!

Sounds

Remember that playlist that you made for your labour and birth? It may need a tweak here and there, but revisiting music that makes you feel happy and in love will help with those all-important endorphins as your hormones fluctuate post-birth. There is also lots of evidence to suggest that babies are responsive to sounds that they became familiar with while growing in the womb, so continuing to hear your voice or regularly played songs will be likely to calm and reassure your baby once they are Earthside. You could also look for yoga or meditation playlists on music platforms like Spotify – there are so many good ones out there and it can be nice to switch off to music you're not so familiar with from time to time.

Sights

When we think about what our baby has been used to in the safety of our womb, we can assume that bright lighting is going to be the ultimate contrast. With this in mind, aim to keep visual surroundings dimly lit and comforting. Lamps, fairy lights and tea lights can be a brilliant alternative to brightly lit rooms, and will be more cosy and relaxing for you, too. I'd also really recommend getting a rechargeable LED touch lamp to keep next to your bed and/or in baby's room for those middle-of-the-night meetings you'll be having a lot of right now.

As a positive addition to what you're seeing, remember that the power of affirmations doesn't stop with birth, and having visual reminders of what a great job you're doing can give you such a great boost emotionally in those early days. Dot affirmation cards around where you're going to see them regularly – this is a good one to get your partner involved with too!

I consciously create an environment that feels safe and secure

FEEDING YOUR BABY

One of the most talked-about topics of new parenthood, and one that will have a big impact on your fourth trimester, is how you choose to feed your baby. Up until birth, your amazing placenta nourished and sustained your baby and met of all their nutritional requirements without any effort on their part; so feeding on the outside world is naturally going to be a transition, and more importantly a learning curve, for both you and your baby. Neither of you have done this before, and whether you are breast- or bottle-feeding, or a bit of both, there are lots of things you can do to make this journey a more positive and empowering one.

The most important thing to do is research and explore your choices around how you are going to feed your baby, and then align this with your intuition and personal preferences. You may have heard the term 'fed is best' bandied around a lot in recent years, and while I understand the sentiment behind this phrase, wouldn't it be wonderful if we were supporting and empowering women to realise that actually, *informed* and *supported* is best?

Feeding your baby is about more than milk, and your choices are likely to have an impact on the health and well-being of both you and your baby, emotionally and physically.

Breastfeeding is of course the most natural food source for your baby, but that doesn't make it everyone's choice or reality. Breastfeeding can be incredible, but it is also demanding, physically and emotionally, and it's a whole new skill that you will need to learn with your baby when they are born. Bottle-feeding can bring its own challenges too. Every feeding journey will have its obstacles, and it's being able to navigate those calmly and with confidence that will feel most rewarding. However you decide to feed your baby, it's important that you feel really well clued-up and supported, and ready to bend or reroute with any unexpected turns your feeding journey takes along the way.

In my experience, I think it's important that however you are going to feed your baby, you find a local lactation consultant whose expertise and support you can access as and when you need to. Even if you're planning on combined or exclusive bottle-feeding, a lactation consultant will be able to provide useful information and support regarding paced/responsive feeding, expressing, and even about things like how to manage feeding your baby when or if you are returning to work. Breastfeeding education is notoriously poor in the UK (which correlates predictably with our low breastfeeding rates), so I think it's crucial that you don't rely solely on the information that appears before you in a two-page leaflet, and instead, learn about the intricacies and the nature of breastfeeding as early on as possible in your journey. The La Leche League has some brilliant resources, and there are likely to be local milk spots (a place where you can drop in to feed your baby and/or get advice on doing so) or community-run feeding groups, too – again, the more you know about these things the easier they will be to access when your baby arrives. Similarly, we mustn't assume that bottle-feeding is going to be the easier option, as it can take some getting used to for everyone too.

When I had my first son in 2010, I honestly didn't give breastfeeding a second thought. I assumed it would come naturally and be easy, and our two-hour NCT breastfeeding workshop 'confirmed' this. And then my baby was born. Wow. What a shock that was. I'm honestly not lying when I say I genuinely believed babies fed three times a day and that there was nothing more to it than bringing them to the breast. I couldn't have been more wrong and I found it to be the most disorientating and relentless hurdle to motherhood. I resentfully breastfed for five months, hating and dreading every feed in equal parts, and only enjoyed feeding my baby when I switched to a bottle thereafter.

Fast-forward eight years and I knew that breastfeeding was something I wanted to learn a lot more about this time round. I met with my local lactation consultant and she spent hours talking me through the science behind breastfeeding, the art of supply and demand, positioning, newborn stomach sizes, age-appropriate food and sleep behaviours, troubleshooting, health and immunity benefits, gut physiology, milk make-up and its links to newborn sleep. My mind was BLOWN. I can't even believe I managed to feed for a week with my first son, let alone five months, when I compared how differently I felt going into my second baby's arrival.

It's not that feeding was necessarily *easier* second time round, it's more that I was better prepared and more empowered to make the decisions that felt right for me and my family at the time. And therefore I was more able to put in place the space and support I would need to have a happier and more fulfilling feeding journey. I knew that along the way those same doubts I had the first time round would creep in, but I also knew I had the professional and personal support in place to work through them, make changes, and continue to learn along the way. For me, the physical and emotional benefits of choosing to breastfeed outweighed the freedom I knew I'd be sacrificing, but it's important to acknowledge that this won't be the case for everyone and that's okay. Mum's mental health comes top of the priority lists here, and as long as you are making informed decisions based on what feels right for you and your family, then Mama, you are doing the PERFECT job.

Remember, too, that you can also take the time to prepare to have a really positive bottle-feeding journey. A lot of women will feel really comforted by knowing to the millilitre how much milk her baby is getting, and by partners getting to share the feeds and those special moments of bonding, so all of these things can be considered when choosing how you're going to feed your baby.

There are lots of lovely ways to incorporate closeness and intimacy into however you're feeding your baby. Below are some things to consider whichever path you take. If you're bottle-feeding your baby and other people will feed them sometimes, it can be really nice to involve them in your feeding ideas and habits, so that your baby is getting fed in a consistent way, and enjoying those special, quiet moments whoever's arms they are in.

Feed in a place that's quiet and consistent

In those early days and weeks, it can be really reassuring for your baby to have calm associations with feeding. Feed your baby somewhere quiet and dark where they won't be distracted by what's going on around them. If you're out and about, you could consider using a muslin or feeding cover to create that safe space on the go.

Centre yourself before a feed

Whether you are breast- or bottle-feeding your baby, it is the time when your baby is at their closest to you. A newborn baby will always co-regulate their breathing with their caregiver's, so before you feed your baby, take a moment to notice your breathing, relax your shoulders, inhale peace and exhale tension. This is a great time to practise your Calm Breath activity (see page 33). If you're breastfeeding, this can also really help with any let-down discomfort when baby latches; and your baby will feed more soundly if you're more comfortable, too.

Skin and eye contact

Feeding, right now, is one of the most important things happening for your baby and it's a great time to capitalise on the opportunity for intimacy and attachment. Holding your baby close to your skin boosts the production of oxytocin and endorphins, which are the hormones that encourage bonding, and it's also a lovely opportunity to gaze lovingly at your baby and let them know that they have everything they need!

Take your time

Whether you're giving your baby the bottle or breast, it's important to go at your baby's speed and not try to rush the process. Remember that a newborn's tummy is tiny and they're still getting used to the sucking reflex, so go slow and allow lots of time for each feed. Giving your baby regular breaks to acclimatise and bring up any gas means they'll be less likely to suffer discomfort afterwards and therefore be more likely to have a sounder sleep. On page 104 we're going to look at newborn stomach sizes in more detail, and this will really help you to understand why little, often and baby-led is key.

I make informed decisions that feel right for me and my family

ACTIVITY

PRESENCE PEBBLES

This activity will require a little forward planning and, if you're reading this in advance of your baby's birth, it makes for a lovely baby shower activity. Alternatively, it can be a nice way to involve other children, or even just a calming sensory exercise to enjoy by yourself.

These presence pebbles are very easy to make, and you're going to use them as anchoring cues whenever and however you're feeding your baby.

1. Collect a handful of stones (start with four or five – you can always add to your collection!)
2. Wash them in warm soapy water, and let them dry thoroughly. You can scrub them with an old toothbrush

to get the dirt off, and sand off any gritty parts with a nail file or sandpaper.

3. While you're waiting for them to dry, think of some affirmations or short positive statements that you might need to hear when you're feeding your baby. They could be things like:

   I am giving my baby what they need
   I enjoy feeding my baby
   We work together to make feeding great
   I am on my own feeding journey
   I relax and enjoy feeding my baby
   My baby and I are healthy and strong
   I follow my instincts

4. Using acrylic paints or pens, write one of your statements onto each stone and decorate however you wish. If you're not using a self-sealing acrylic paint, coat with a sealer spray and again, allow to dry thoroughly.
5. Keep your stones in a small bag and in a place that's easy to access when you're feeding. During a feed, pull out one of your stones and focus your energy on the positive reminder it offers you.

Focusing on a presence pebble during a feed will mean your breathing slows, along with your heart rate, which your baby will pick up on and respond to positively. It will also help alleviate discomfort and make each feed a calmer and more enjoyable experience for you both.

If you'd like to try out your ideas before painting your pebbles, you can do it here…

I follow my instincts

I enjoy feeding my baby

My baby and I are healthy and strong

NURTURING YOURSELF

The birth of your baby doesn't end with them leaving your body. You've spent a whole nine months (maybe more!) watching your body change to accommodate and nourish this little baby inside of you, and now that they are here, your body continues the hard work. Birth is a bit like the sandwich filling of becoming a mother. You have all this time to prepare – mentally and physically – for birthing and meeting your baby, and then when your baby is here, your body and mind begin their journey in adapting to motherhood.

We've already explored some of the physical discomforts you may be experiencing after the birth of your baby (see page 15), and just as you navigated the aches and pains you may have experienced then and during pregnancy, try to be kind, nurturing and patient with your body as it recovers from the incredible work it's been doing, and continues to do. You may be sore, tender and sensitive after birth, and it's important that you are kind and go gently (and lovingly) with your new mother's body.

Something I consider to be a bit of a golden nugget of wisdom when it comes to the post-partum period is to go as slowly as you possibly can. After your baby's birth, I would highly recommend spending a week in bed. I know that in a culture that glorifies busy, this suggestion may sound ridiculously decadent, but really, it was hands-down the single best thing I did second time round, and made such a profound difference to my physical and emotional recovery. In comparison to my first experience eight years prior, it improved the way I bonded with my baby, how we established breastfeeding, my physical recovery post second C-section, and even my memory of those magical first few days (it remains an absolute and total blur with my first!).

Spending a week in bed means that you can mostly be unclothed – ideal for establishing feeding, bonding and all of that skin-to-skin we've talked about – and you will find it so much easier to learn and respond to your baby's feeding cues than if you're trying to do five other things at the same time. It also means you can nap intermittently, which will make the nights, when baby is often hungrier and needs feeding more, easier to cope with. Honestly, the time and presence you can put in here will make your life so much easier going forward. Think of it as an investment in your future self. You have nowhere to be other than here. A slow and still period immediately post-partum will also allow your body to physically heal more quickly, meaning you'll feel stronger and more robust as time goes on.

Note: If you're a few weeks or months into your motherhood journey and you're reading this wishing you'd done it, or thinking it's too late, it's really not! I often talk to mums about the value of a belated baby bubble, and believe me, it can be incredible! Check out the Belated Baby Bubble activity on page 257.

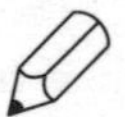

ACTIVITY

NUGGETS OF NOURISHMENT

In the early days of life with your baby, the idea of nurturing yourself can feel near impossible, but I think this fourth trimester is about expectation management and adjusting the boundaries of your life to reflect your current reality. While yoga practice, lunch dates and massages might seem a way off, I want to give you some ideas for nurturing yourself when time, energy

and logistics aren't as they used to be and the days are topsy-turvy. Think of this in a very basic way, almost as if you are meeting the needs of your small child. Ask yourself the following questions.

Am I warm enough?

Am I hungry or thirsty?

Am I tired?

Do I feel physically and emotionally comfortable?

You will constantly be directing these questions at your little one, but try to find a moment each day where you can ask them of yourself, too. Bookmark this page as a place to come back to when you're feeling depleted or like you just need a breather from the demands of life with a newborn. The more you can get accustomed to checking in with yourself in this way now, the more likely you are to continue this simple practice of self-care long into your motherhood journey. Isn't it lovely to think you could still be asking yourself these loving questions when your children are teenagers?!

Because it's often easy to underestimate the benefits of self-nourishment, I want you to use the space on pages 69–70 to log how you feel before doing the activities I've suggested, and then again afterwards. Consider your experience of the following sensations: mental clarity, emotional presence, physical comfort. Give your experience of them a rating out of ten before and afterwards. Once we realise these activities are of value to our physical and emotional state, we are more likely to draw on them again in times of stress or fatigue. Our mind remembers when something feels good, and will look for it again when we feel in need.

TAKE A BATH

When your baby is sleeping, or if you have a partner or friend who's willing to provide an hour's worth of cuddles, run yourself a warm bath and use some oils or bath salts to make it a more nourishing experience (although if you have a wound or stitches, check with your midwife or care provider first that this will be safe). Listen to a podcast or some relaxing music to help lighten your mind and give you a breather from care-mode.

TAKE OFF YOUR SHOES

This might sound like a strange one, but if you have a garden and the weather is on your side, take off your shoes and stand on the grass for ten minutes. Connecting with nature and feeling the warm grass underneath you can offer such a welcome sense of relaxation and grounding. If you don't have access to grass, put your feet in a bowl of warm water for twenty minutes – you can even do this while feeding or holding your baby, and it can serve as a great recharge.

PHONE OR TEXT A FRIEND

If you're having a wobble or feeling tired and depleted, lean on the energy of a good friend and tell them how you feel. Taking a moment to offload and decompress can feel like a huge weight has been lifted from the mental load of motherhood, especially in those early days when your world can feel so small.

FEED YOURSELF, TOO

When we're busy meeting the needs of a newborn, it can be easy to overlook our most basic needs. It's so important that new mums are getting nourished from the inside out, so don't underestimate the boost that can come from eating a warm, satisfying meal. You deserve – and more importantly – need it!

NAP. ALWAYS NAP

Before I had kids there was no way I could have napped in the day. In fact, even when I had my first son I resisted because I felt there was too much to do. Fast forward eight years and I'd learned that my emotional experience was directly related to how much sleep I was getting and how rested I felt, and that it is actually the fuel of mothers. The physical demands of motherhood are so much more intense than anything you will have been used to. Napping when your baby does (especially in these early weeks and months) has the power to profoundly improve your entire experience. It's not being lazy, it's keeping your tank topped up, and this is what these months should be all about. If you have trouble napping, even closing your eyes and listening to the short guided meditation you'll have access to with this book (see page 7) can bring about a renewed sense of energy and peace.

Ultimately, remember that by looking after yourself you are looking after your baby.

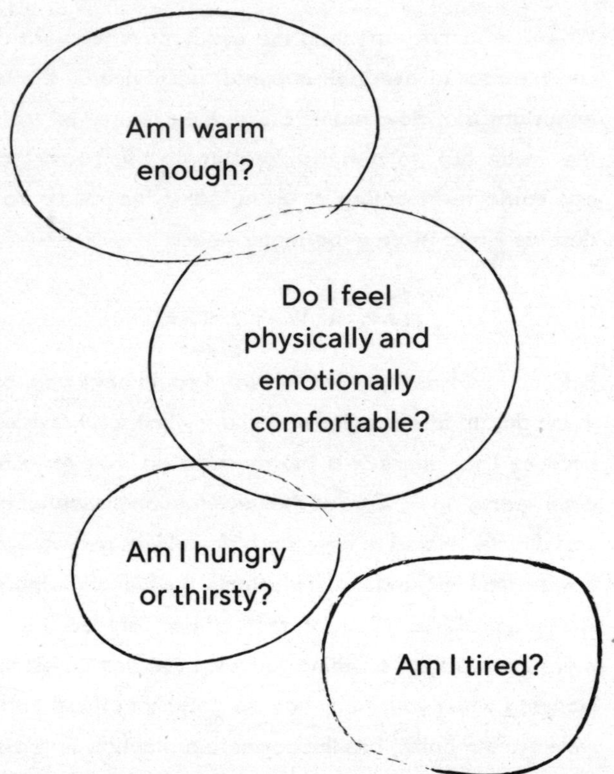

Self-care and nourishment are not luxuries – they provide space for the emotional and physical availability demanded by your little one, and will help you to find calmness and joy amid the intensity of this new reality.

NURTURING YOUR NETWORK (AND LETTING THEM NURTURE YOU!)

We've already touched on this idea that when a new baby is expected, it's natural for extended families to want in on the action from day one, but it's really important to remember that you get to make the rules here – especially for the duration of your fourth trimester. This is your baby, and your experience of parenthood, and it's vital that, either before or immediately after your baby arrives, you create some boundaries for the immediate postnatal period and talk to your nearest and dearest about them.

First, you don't want to be dealing with the anxiety that your whole network might descend on you the moment you've had your first shower, and second, it's a good way to remove the pressure of having (potentially) difficult conversations when you're trying to bond with your newborn. Having this conversation ahead of your baby's arrival means everyone's clear on what you want/need; but if you're holding your baby and realising you haven't done that yet, then it can be a good job to share with your partner or support network, who can let everyone know how and when they can be involved. This means that you can relax, knowing that everyone will be on the same page and that introducing your baby more widely can be a calmer affair.

Of course though, don't feel like you have to commit to maintaining these rules if your feelings change over those first few days and weeks – they are just there as boundaries and you are in charge. If you suddenly feel like you want some support around, and your mum, sister or close friend would be a big help with that, then you're allowed to bend your own rules – you are in the driving seat here! Think of it more as a kind of cloak of protection that means the only person you are looking after is your baby – not other people.

We've talked about the breadth of emotions that the immediate postnatal period can bring with it, and they are inevitably easier to navigate when you're not trying to put on a brave face or entertain other people.

> The feelings and emotions that are born with your baby deserve honouring. They are here to teach you something, to ignite places deep inside your heart and soul, and to switch you on for the emotional landscape of motherhood.

It's well worth remembering, too, if you have a partner, that (depending on the generosity – or even existence – of their parental leave) these first few days and weeks are likely to be an incredibly sacred time for them and your baby to get to know each other. Often, when you are descended upon by lots of friends and family, your partner's leave can turn into two weeks of tidying up and making tea when it could be spent helping you to heal and bonding with baby. There will be so much time ahead for others to meet your little one, but your partner is unlikely to get this solid block of time to be around you both again, and that's really something to treasure and protect.

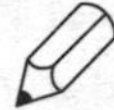

ACTIVITY

ASK FOR WHAT YOU NEED

Many of us don't feel comfortable asking for what we truly need, so in this exercise we're going to make it that little bit easier by writing things down rather than leaving ourselves exposed and on the spot. While we've talked about leaning on the support of your network in those first few days of life with your baby (see page 27), it's brilliant if you can continue to lean on them during your fourth trimester (and beyond). Getting this stuff down on paper (or on the space on pages 77–78) also helps us to bring it to the front of our mind and work out what's important, and what's not.

Start by thinking about what kind of things make you feel better and more at ease. What could people do to help you, support you, and make your life easier? Most people really WANT to help, but often don't know how (or do it in a way that may not feel right for us), so by getting a clearer sense of it in your own mind, you'll be able to communicate it more easily to others. Here's a bit more on the ideas we talked about in The First 48 Hours:

FOOD: The one thing I wanted in the early days with my newborns was good, warm food. Unfortunately, I didn't turn out to be one of those people who got organised with batch-cooking ahead of baby's arrival, so instead I relied heavily on the kind gestures of family and friends who were looking after us in this way.

That said, you don't necessarily want to end up with a fridge full of mince-based meals (lasagne, chilli – you know the score, the comfort food classics that we can pull from the top of our head), so why not do the legwork for your loved ones and source some simple, nourishing recipes that they could cook for you. Think tasty soups, stews, vegetable bakes and wholesome pies: things that are easy to heat and yummy to eat. Talk to them before your baby arrives about how they can help you after the birth, and ask if they'd be happy to bring or send a meal when they come and meet your little one for the first time. Providing them with a new recipe will expand their repertoire too, and suddenly everyone's a winner!

Food and nourishment are such loving gestures, and this is one that you can embrace as a way of supporting each other within your family or friendship circle over the years to come. There will always be someone who needs support at different times in their lives, and this is a brilliant way to initiate that cycle of taking care of one another.

HOUSEHOLD JOBS: This is another brilliant one. Think of simple household chores that you might not feel up to doing when you've just had your baby (this is even more relevant if you know you're having a C-section), write them down on little pieces of paper and pop them in a jar. They could be things like: Fifteen minutes of ironing, stacking/unstacking the dishwasher, taking the bins out, cleaning the bathroom, running the hoover around, etc, etc. Let your family and friends know that there will be a little-jobs jar on offer when they come and meet your baby, and how grateful you'd be if they could dip in and pick a pot-luck job during their visit. You'll get a job done that's actually helpful, and they'll feel great for being able to support you in that way. If you have other children or pets, it can also be wise to see who can help you out with school runs/dog walks in the week or so after your baby has arrived.

If there are people who are less able or who you wouldn't necessarily feel comfortable asking for this level of help from, you could ask for simpler support. Maybe they could pick you up some milk and a packet of biscuits on their way over, collect a parcel or pop something in the postbox for you on their way back home.

There are also some ground rules you'll want to think about. For example, are you happy for others to hold your baby? Some mums are grateful for an extra pair of arms so that they can grab a nap or take a breather, but some prefer for baby not to be passed around in those early days – both completely valid! It's sensible to ask family and friends to visit only if they're in good health, and to wash their hands when they arrive. Also think about how long you're happy for a visit to be, and don't be afraid to set that boundary so that others are clear about what's okay.

When you feel like you've got your ideas together, you could tie it all up in an email or WhatsApp message so that everyone knows what to expect when the time comes. Keep it warm and friendly – remember that asking for what you need is not indulgent or unreasonable, it's a way for everyone to be clear on the boundaries of your sacred postnatal period, and how they can be warmly and actively involved in that.

It could be something like:

> *To our awesome friends and family. We know you are so excited about our little one's arrival, and we can't wait for you to meet them. We really want to have the most calm and special time getting to know our new baby, so we'd ask for your love and practical support while we find our way:*
>
> - *When you get here, please text, as the doorbell might wake a sleeping baby*
> - *Please wash your hands and take off your shoes*
> - *If you're not feeling well let's reschedule*
> - *Mum is probably busy feeding baby, so a hand around the house would be gratefully received. Pick a pot-luck job from our jar – none of them take more than fifteen minutes, we promise!*
> - *[Continue to add your own]*
>
> *Thanks for your support, love and understanding – it means a lot to us!*

Reciprocal respect and compassion with the people around you – your partner, friends, family and colleagues – will make your ongoing experience of motherhood easier, happier and more relaxed.

MEETING MUMS

I think it's also worth mentioning here that you may have a real or virtual group of new mum friends who you've met through antenatal classes or similar. Often when we're pregnant we can spend a lot of time thinking about who we're going to lean on when our baby arrives, and this can be a big part of what prompts us to attend antenatal groups like NCT or similar. It's easy to put a lot of expectation into these people instantly becoming our ready-made friendship circle, and it's great when that happens, but remember it's definitely not always the case, and it's far from the be-all and end-all of your opportunities for social support.

If you have been fortunate enough to meet some like-minded souls, you may well have a WhatsApp group or similar going to facilitate some camaraderie and conversation about what you're all going through. Hopefully you and the women you connect with will create a safe and judgement-free space, but it's really important to remember that everyone deals with things differently and you're unlikely to know enough about these women to have the full picture of their coping mechanisms. While some will lay everything bare and say it how it is, some might feel better keeping their cards close to their chest and suggesting that their journey is unfolding problem-free. Share what you are comfortable with and let your intuition lead you on who you feel safe with. Try to avoid comparisons and remember that you have nothing to prove.

If the women you've met through your groups aren't your cup of tea, that's okay too. This isn't your only opportunity to make friends, and trust me when I say you'll meet the right people at the right time for the right reasons. It can often be really reassuring to have even the simplest of connections with other women going through similar moments to you, whether that's a virtual hello on the night feeds or a slow stroll around the park with some understanding company, but these are the very first laps of this new circuit, and you can refine what you're looking for as the weeks, months and years go by.

We'll talk more about really finding your tribe a little later on, but you can hop forward to page 182 if you are eager to read more right now.

I nurture myself so that I can nurture my baby

RIDING THE EMOTIONAL ROLLERCOASTER

We've talked a lot about the huge spectrum of emotions you might be feeling in the first 48 hours, and of course that's likely to extend well into your fourth trimester. Our emotions tend to be especially heightened soon after we've given birth, especially as our hormones surge, but over the next few weeks and months, they will remain a big part of your postnatal experience. Some days you will feel absolutely amazing – like you're floating on cloud nine and high on love – while others may feel like way more of a struggle. Some days things will go your way, and some days they won't. This is completely normal and I will be sharing lots of tips and tricks with you here for how to become more at ease with the flow of what can, at times, feel like an emotional rollercoaster.

If you have had a difficult or traumatic birth experience, I think that processing this can play a huge part in riding the emotional waves of the fourth trimester. I'll be talking about this in more detail on page 88 but please know that there is lots of support out there for helping you to overcome and heal from a birth that you feel is affecting your postnatal experience. Your feelings are always valid, you are not alone, and you can heal.

BABY BLUES OR POSTNATAL DEPRESSION?

You may well have heard from your midwife or health visitor, or from other mothers, about the 'baby blues', which most women will experience at some point during the week or two following their baby's birth. In the first couple of weeks of your baby's life, it's really normal to experience mood swings, feel low, teary or mildly depressed; not surprising given everything you are dealing with. Sleep deprivation and the weight of responsibility when you bring your baby home can be overwhelming, and brings up all sorts of emotions that you may not be expecting.

The baby blues is triggered by all of this in combination with your fluctuating hormones, your physical recovery from birth, and your milk coming in around day three. This is a completely normal part of the early postnatal period and the majority of new mums will say they've experienced these baby blues to some degree. Remember that feeling tearful and overwhelmed doesn't mean you're doing anything wrong, and that it is a natural part of our hormonal adaptation to motherhood. These feelings are likely to be at their strongest in week one, and then taper off during week two, although this will vary from woman to woman.

When you accept this as a normal part of the post-partum period and know that it comes from a place of your body continuing to work hard, you will find yourself in a better place to nurture yourself through it, and offer yourself some kindness and compassion as you navigate this new territory.

Another good reason to protect your first couple of weeks from lots of visitors is so that you feel safe and comfortable to lean into this rollercoaster of emotions without feeling like you have to put on a constantly happy face. It can be really helpful to have one or two close companions (maybe a partner or a close friend) who you can talk to when you feel low, and who will know how to make you feel heard, loved and well supported.

For some women, these baby blues don't taper off and the feelings of exhaustion, despair and sadness seem to grow stronger. If this happens, or you can't feel your low mood lifting, you may be suffering from postnatal depression (PND), which is a more serious problem and one that you can and should get professional support for.

Postnatal depression can often be disguised as the baby blues in the early weeks of your baby's life, and this is why your midwife will spend time talking about your emotional recovery and how you're feeling in your postnatal appointments at home or at your local children's centre. It's so important to be honest with your midwife – you can trust them completely and they will not judge you at all if you say you're worried or scared. Lots of women worry that they'll be seen as unfit, or that their baby will be taken away, but this is not the case – your midwife and care providers will give you the help and support you need so that you can feel better and enjoy your journey.

Common symptoms of PND include heightened mood swings that continue beyond the baby blues, feelings of deep sadness, hopelessness, insomnia and irritability. Some women will even feel suicidal or that they are unable to care for their baby. PND can also include feelings of guilt, despair, worthlessness and withdrawal from those who love you, so if you are feeling this way then know that you are not alone and you can and will get better – you just have to ask for help. There are lots of avenues for talking therapy or medication that can be explored with your care provider if you're feeling unable to cope or think your mental health is suffering after the birth of your baby. Being proactive in seeking out this support is really courageous, and so beneficial to both you and your baby.

If you have a partner, it can be very useful to talk to them about these elements of the postnatal period so that they can help to support and safeguard you in an informed and compassionate way. The more we think of the postnatal period as an emotional journey as well as a physical one, the more equipped we are to navigate the trickier bits – together.

You already know from those first couple of days with your baby that learning to become comfortable with whatever feelings arise can really help you to ride all these new emotional waves. What I'd invite you to do is continue considering what these feelings might look and feel like for you over the coming months with your baby; and perhaps consider it in a bit more depth now that you are getting used to what your new reality looks like. Even though they may feel overwhelming and uncomfortable at times, the truth is that you've actually felt lots of these things before and have come through the other side. So know that you can feel them again now and thrive. Acknowledging this will help what you're feeling to become more tangible and manageable and help to lessen any uneasiness or sense of the unknown.

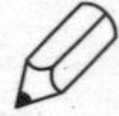

ACTIVITY

GRAB THE FEELINGS FIRST

This activity is about grabbing hold of emotions before they grab hold of you. By identifying and acknowledging the wide range of normal human emotions we all experience throughout our lives, we can lessen the hold they have over us and reduce any feelings of negativity we have towards them. It's important to remember that there are no 'good' or 'bad' emotions or feelings; just our individual responses to challenging situations. Allowing the space to acknowledge whatever you're feeling will help you feel better equipped to face them if and when they show up again.

In the space overleaf, have a go at writing down some of the emotions you might feel (or have already felt) in the days and weeks following your baby's birth. You can use the ones we talked about on page 21 or add others that spring to mind for you now (or that you've experienced before, if this isn't your first baby).

Then consider how these emotions really make you feel, both physically and mentally. What helps you to cope with them when they arise? How you can get better at embracing them as you settle into motherhood and learn more about your baby? What do you need to help you through each emotion – what will make you feel supported? If this proves tricky, try thinking back to a time when you've experienced this emotion in the past, and identify what helped you process it then.

For example:

> **SADNESS:** *When I feel sad, I want to be held and reassured. Sadness can leave me feeling doubtful or hopeless and it can sometimes lead me to think everything is a catastrophe. I don't want to be sociable when I feel sad, and only want the people I feel safest with around me. Sometimes I try to put on a brave face or distract myself from feeling sad, but that can make me feel physically uncomfortable and prolong it, so it's better if I allow myself to have a cry as a way to let the sadness out of my body. When I'm able to feel it and let it out, I feel calmer and more at ease, and the sadness passes more quickly.*

This makes me think back to when I had my first son in 2010. I felt very overwhelmed and sometimes just felt like crying. Initially, I kept resisting the urge to cry by distracting myself, or even convincing myself that I 'shouldn't' cry, but the feeling never went away and, in hindsight, felt way worse inside than it did when it eventually came out. A friend of mine suggested that I watched a nostalgic or soppy film, or something with a few tear-jerker moments, and oh my goodness, it made such a difference! Whenever I felt emotional, I would sit on the sofa with my baby and put on something that I knew would get the tears flowing, and the relief and release I felt just from having a good cry was immense! It didn't mean I was getting anything wrong, or not enjoying my baby, it was just the simple fact that I had all of this emotion bottled up that needed an outlet – and gosh, did that outlet make me feel better!

Exploring your feelings in this way – considering how they make you feel physically and mentally – may have a similar effect on you, taking you back to a time when you happened upon the tools to better process your feelings. Revisit this activity often, because I bet you'll be surprised by how many lightbulb moments you can identify and use to your advantage in motherhood. Also, don't feel like you have to complete this activity in one go. It's something you can come back to and add to when you feel like; or keep it running as a work-in-progress.

PROCESSING YOUR BIRTH EXPERIENCE

In the overwhelm of the first few days and weeks with your new baby, you may find that the birth disappears from your mind temporarily, only to reappear a week or two later when you start to find your groove and your hormones are beginning to settle.

Maybe you had a great birth; maybe you had a traumatic one. Maybe it was neither, or somewhere in between. Whatever your birth was like, the memory (whether conscious or not) will stay with you on a deep level, and it can be incredibly helpful and cathartic to give space to processing how you felt and then acknowledging, celebrating or healing from the way it unfolded.

ACTIVITY

WRITING YOUR BIRTH STORY

Writing your birth story is one of those things that many women really want to do, but never get round to. It can fall to the bottom of the list, only for you to find that when you finally get the chance, your memories are blurred.

If possible, I'd really encourage you to jot down notes about your birth as soon as you can. It can be a work-in-progress, and something you work up as the weeks go by, but do try to get snapshots of these memories down while they are fresh and vivid.

Think of it as something that's for your eyes only, so that you can write openly and honestly about your experience. You can start with the tangible things like the date, time, where you were when labour started and how your labour unfolded. You could include things like the songs you listened to, what the people who looked after you were like, and then delve deeper into how you felt and what your experience felt like.

Try to capture how you felt when you met your baby, and what happened afterwards. These memories are likely to be incredibly precious and visceral, and having an eternal log of them will be something you're so grateful for in the months and years to come.

You may find that this activity brings up lots of emotion for you, but remember this isn't a bad thing. If the emotions are there, they will affect you whether you acknowledge them or not, so an activity like this is a way of letting them breathe.

HEALING AFTER TRAUMA

If you had a difficult or traumatic birth, you may not feel like you can do the birth story activity yet, and that's okay too. The most important thing to remember is that a frightening or upsetting birth experience is never your fault. Sometimes in birth, things fall out of our hands or we aren't treated in a way that felt empowering, and we are left trying to salvage what happened while trying to 'be grateful' that our baby is okay. Please hear this: you can be grateful that your baby is okay and still grieve an experience that wasn't as you envisaged, hoped or prepared for. Your feelings are valid and there are lots of really nurturing avenues for helping you to process Post Traumatic Stress Disorder (PTSD – anxiety specifically caused by distressing or frightening events) or birth trauma.

Talking therapy

We've touched on the signposts for postnatal depression and low mood on page 81, but again, it's really important that you talk to your midwife (or make an appointment to speak to your GP) if the experience of your birth is affecting how you feel on a daily basis. Most hospitals and NHS trusts offer a birth debriefing or birth reflection service free of charge. You can ask your midwife or health visitor about this and they will retrieve your notes and invite you in for an appointment to go through them with you. This can often be really helpful in getting a better understanding of what happened, and giving yourself a chance to process and reflect on how you felt. You don't necessarily need to have had an overtly or physically traumatic birth to be suffering with birth trauma – it can be triggered by the way you felt you were treated or spoken to, and a debriefing will really help you to identify these elements and get a better idea for how you can move forward.

If you can afford private therapy, I would highly recommend it as you'll get support more quickly, but it is available through the NHS too. If private therapy seems financially inaccessible, it's also worth speaking to local therapists to see if they offer concessions for daytime or off-peak appointments, or look for someone who is expanding their training and experience and offering discounted rates. They key is in finding someone you feel safe and comfortable with, so don't be afraid to speak to them on the phone or in person first for an initial consultation. To find a qualified therapist in your area, visit the British Association for Counselling and Psychotherapy at www.bacp.co.uk.

3-Step Rewind Technique

The 3-Step Rewind Technique for birth trauma is an incredibly effective way of processing birth trauma in the space of two or three sessions. It involves three stages of therapeutic work with a qualified professional: deep relaxation; recalling your birth in a specific way while feeling safe and secure; and then imagining coping in the future and responding differently to how things unfolded and its emotional effects. To find a 3-Step Rewind Technique therapist in your area, visit www.traumaticbirthrecovery.com.

Emotional Freedom Technique (EFT)

EFT is a relatively new form of therapy that draws from theories of acupuncture, NLP (neuro-linguistic programming), thought field therapy and energy healing. In my experience, it can be hugely beneficial to those processing emotional distress or overcoming trauma, and what's particularly useful with EFT is that once you have been taught how to tap into it, it becomes a simple form of self-administered therapy. Many women I've worked with have used this and the 3-Step Rewind Technique to overcome birth trauma, with really profound effects.

Ultimately, if you are suffering then know that there is help out there, and you are always stronger than you realise. Here are three daily reminders to help you heal and find your inner resilience:

1. I am not alone
2. My experiences are valid
3. There is help and support out there to help me heal

EMBRACING THE TOPSY-TURVY NATURE OF THESE EARLY DAYS

So now that we've talked about your baby's needs and the spectrum of emotions that might be whizzing around in those precious first days and weeks, let's turn our attention to what life might actually *look* like once you're back at home with your baby.

In my experience, and having taken very different immediate post-natal approaches with my two babies, the key to a calm and enjoyable baby bubble is zero expectation and the kindness to prioritise yourself completely. Before you know it, you're going to be out and about walking in the park, meeting friends, nestling down in coffee shops, showing your baby off, or attending singing groups or classes, but you will never, ever, go back to these first few days and weeks.

It is a tiny and unique pocket of time that, if savoured, can really build the robust and resilient foundations on which you can thrive and venture back out into the world.

When you bring a new baby into your home, a lot of things change. There is a lot of new 'stuff' adorning your kitchen/floor/stairs/side tables all of a sudden and I know that for a lot of people, it can bring about feelings of real unease; and that's understandable. For however many years, you've been solely (or jointly) responsible for what your home looks and feels like, and then all of a sudden this tiny little human appears who not only seems to accumulate a lot of paraphernalia, but also does a lot of, shall we say, leaking? There's wee, poo, sick, milk, along with the other mysterious bodily fluids that you inevitably end up discovering at three o'clock in the morning.

It's safe to say that things are going to feel pretty topsy-turvy right now, and while that might not be traditionally identifiable as your comfort zone, remember that it's temporary and that it's okay. Looking after a newborn baby is absolutely and completely a full-time job. In the nine months you've been growing them, your unseen work has been sustaining them 24/7, and this fourth trimester really is an extension of that. Things at home might feel chaotic, but it's for good reason. There's likely to be an unusual amount of mess, dirty dishes in the sink and weird meals in the middle of the night, but what I'm inviting you to do here is to identify your short-term priorities and embrace the slightly bonkers discombobulation as something sacred and unique to this tiny pocket of time.

Each day I learn and grow as a mother

ACTIVITY

PRIORITY PLATE-SPINNING

When I work with pregnant women and new mums, one of the struggles that comes up a lot is the pressure around keeping on top of things at home. As a self-confessed tidy-freak, I can completely relate to the weight of this anxiety, especially at a time when you know you're likely to be spending a lot of time at home. In a moment I'm going to share with you some helpful tips for finding calm among the chaos in these early weeks, but first, I want you to have a go at this fun and thought-provoking exercise about plate-spinning.

Across the page, you'll see a new mum spinning a lot of plates. That's you. You'll also spot her to-do list. This is a general list, and I want you to add underneath any responsibilities or jobs that apply to you personally. Now I want you to prioritise the plates you're spinning. Label the spinning plates with the jobs you consider to be most important. Do you see the stack of plates on the floor beside her? That's where you're going to add the remaining labels. Those plates aren't smashed, fallen or broken. They're just waiting on the floor until she's ready to take them on.

Thinking of your priorities as changeable can really help to manage feelings of overwhelm in the fourth trimester. It's not that the dishes are never going to get done, it's just that they're not going to get done *right now*.

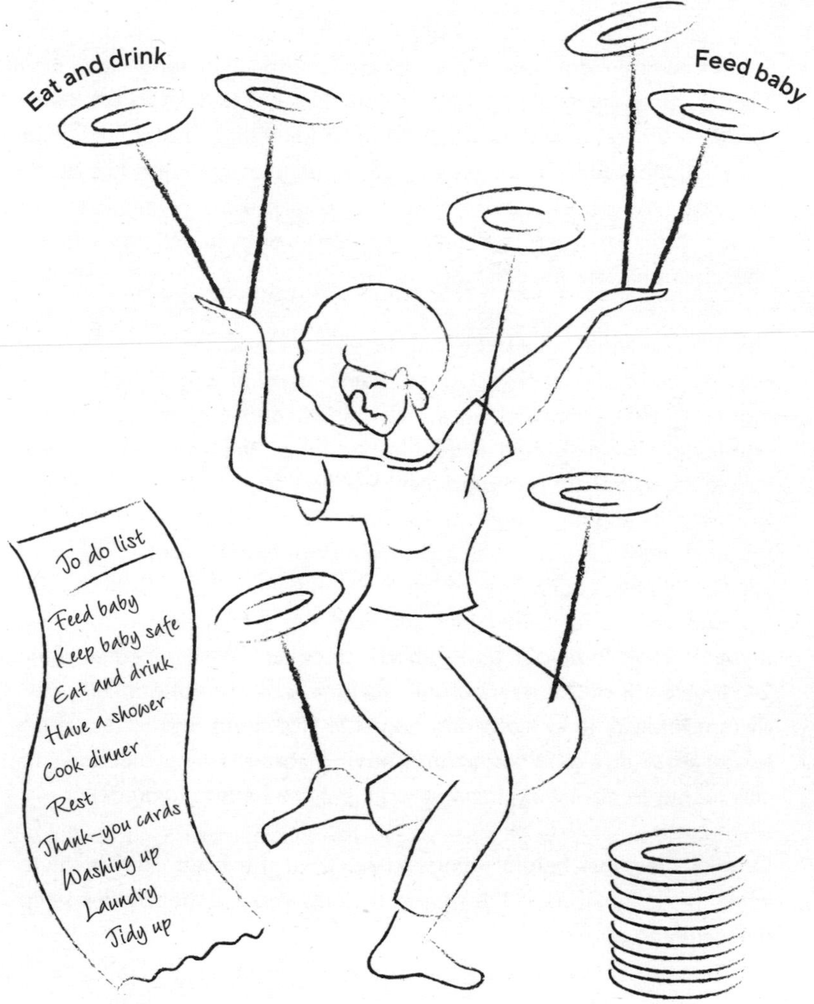

Eat and drink
Feed baby
To do list
Feed baby
Keep baby safe
Eat and drink
Have a shower
Cook dinner
Rest
Thank-you cards
Washing up
Laundry
Tidy up

NAVIGATING YOUR BABY'S SLEEP HABITS (OR LACK OF)

I don't think we can talk about things feeling topsy-turvy right now without mentioning sleep. One of the biggest shocks to all newly 'born' mothers is the unpredictable and testing nature of your baby's sleep habits (or the lack of them), especially during this fourth trimester. We are all very familiar with that million-dollar question: 'how's the baby sleeping?' and the weight of pressure, expectation and disappointment it often brings with it.

The truth is, while your baby might sleep a lot during those first few days as they acclimatise to their Earthside environment, it's something that constantly evolves as your baby does, and it sometimes (okay, often) gets worse before it gets better. Over the next few months, their awake time will gradually increase and they will eventually begin to sleep for slightly longer cycles (more about that later!), but the fourth trimester remains unpredictable and largely dictated by what your baby needs *each day*, rather than internal synchronisation, and this can vary a lot with every day and night that passes for now. Remembering that your baby's body clock isn't yet aligned with the 24-hour clock of this new outside world is really important. This new rhythm takes time to learn and adjust to (for them and for you!), so taking each day as it comes and having some coping mechanisms can be key to not letting this hot topic get the better of you.

One of the most helpful things to keep at the front of your mind while in the trenches of the newborn sleep show is that *babies sleep differently to adults*.

Putting adult-influenced sleep expectations onto babies is a fruitless (and inevitably frustrating) waste of your time and energy. Not only can it lead us to overlooking our little one's calls for help, but it can actually interrupt their natural development towards more mature, age-appropriate sleep patterns when they are ready and able.

While it feels hard and relentless, nurturing your baby's immediate and changing sleep needs in a responsive and accepting way will set you all up for healthier, happier sleep rhythms further down the line. Learning to cope and embrace the erratic nature of your baby's sleep habits over the next twelve weeks is the key to feeling more calm and confident in meeting their needs without losing your mind, so let's look at ways you can do this.

Learning day and night rhythms

One of the most obvious differences between adult and newborn sleep is that while we follow day and night rhythms of being awake and asleep, our babies approach it as an unsegmented 24-hour period, meaning they continue to cycle through being awake and asleep regardless of which part of day or night they're in. This is all down to the circadian rhythm – an internal clock that adults live by, but that babies haven't yet adapted to. The circadian rhythm (otherwise known as our primal or inbuilt sleep/wake cycle) constantly runs in the background of our brains, and moves between sleepiness and alertness at regular intervals.

Without getting too deep on the science (it's a big topic!), our circadian rhythm is affected by our brain activity, hormones, cell regeneration and our daily exposure to light. For example, sunlight helps our body to calibrate its internal clock, while darkness triggers our brain to signal the production of melatonin, the hormone that paves the way for sleep. This is why staring at your bright phone screen or laptop right before bed can prevent you from getting to sleep – you're confusing the information your brain is receiving with regards to light/dark and it can't respond until it works things out.

Interestingly, when babies are still in utero they are linked to this circadian rhythm because maternal melatonin passes through the placenta and so can affect their internal clock. Similarly, their heart rate often speeds up when Mum is active and slows down when she sleeps – such is the intimate, internal influence of maternal hormones during pregnancy. Once a baby is born though, this connection is broken and babies will need to learn to synchronise their cycles all over again, and this typically takes at least twelve weeks, when babies start to produce their own melatonin hormone.

Nurturing your newborn's experience of the circadian rhythm

While trying to implement any kind of routine in the fourth trimester can prove fruitless, there are ways that you can support your newborn in becoming more in sync with day and night. Try exposing them to light for short periods during the day (taking them out for a walk in the buggy, or sitting in a bright room or garden), and then contrasting this with a darker environment when you are winding down for bed. You can also try to reduce stimulation in the evenings – quieter voices, dimmer lights, less movement – as these will slowly become recognisable signposts for night-time.

Sleep thieves and strategies

Hopefully now that you understand a bit more about why babies sleep (or don't) the way they do, you can reframe the reasoning and acknowledge the temporary nature of this time. Having this deeper understanding of what your baby is learning and adapting to can make it less frustrating, but I'm well aware that doesn't take away from the painful realities of sleep deprivation.

I'm going to share with you my five tips for fatigue, which will hopefully keep your cup topped up enough to keep pouring. It's inevitable that some days will just feel un-doable and you'll feel like you're clawing through till bedtime, but I think implementing these easy ideas can help you to feel a little more robust and well equipped when the going gets tough.

1. Don't skip breakfast

With busy, full-on mornings (especially if you have other children to get ready for school etc), it can be easy to feed everyone else and worry about yourself later, but this can have a big impact on your energy and blood sugar levels throughout the day. Start thinking of breakfast as your morning fuel, and if you can't seem to find the time to fit in making something, prepare something the night before. Something like overnight oat jars are easy to make, brilliantly nutritious, and require no prep on busy mornings.

2. Start with a stretch

After a broken night's sleep it's no wonder we wake up feeling stiffer and more tired than when we went to bed. Having a stretch first thing can help to get your circulation going and boost your energy levels quicker than a cup of coffee! Again, it's not something you've got to carve out a separate moment in time for – try stretching while you're brushing your teeth, putting your clothes on, or walking down the stairs.

3. Prepare handy snacks in advance

Much like with breakfast, it can be so easy as new mums to get to the end of the day and realise we've just grazed on cold toast and cake. Now, I very much like a slice of cake and still hold each slice as a cherished memory of those early days, but stock up on some handy snacks that are fuelling you nutritiously too. Lots of companies now make grazing boxes or energy balls; or have a go at whizzing up your own. You can make a massive batch and freeze them (or ask someone else to!) so they'll always be on hand when you feel your energy levels dipping.

4. A soundtrack for your sanity

During both of my babies' first years I would often find that my exhaustion was compounded by the lack of adult voices, music or chatter that I'd been used to in the workplace. Try creating an uplifting playlist of energy-boosting songs that will lift your mood and heart rate, or try listening to a podcast that grabs your attention. It could be anything from comedy to true crime to insightful interviews – anything that will spark your attention and have you feeling less drowsy and more fired up.

5. It's not just naps

You've already heard me bang on about the power of a good nap, but I know it's not always possible. If your baby is asleep, try just sitting on the sofa and closing your eyes for anything from five to twenty minutes for a midday reboot. The itchy eyes of fatigue are horrible, so giving them a well-deserved rest – even if you don't actually snooze – will offer a much-needed dose of comfort.

Cluster feeding and the witching hour

In my personal experience, one of the most difficult and demanding parts of the fourth trimester was the early-evening cluster feeding and its regular link to the witching hour! Honestly, even writing that makes me shudder slightly, such is its bizarre and relentless nature. I'm trying to find the right words to describe this time of day so prevalent in newborns during their first few months on Earth, but actually, the very words *witching hour* really do describe it perfectly (although let's upgrade *hour* to *hours*, okay?).

The witching hours are basically when it feels like your baby has gone from being this serene and sweet little bundle to a fussy, unsoothable, fractious mess in the space of ten minutes. Nothing you do seems to bring them comfort, they seem tired but won't sleep, hungry but won't easily feed, and passing them to someone else just makes it worse. Everything you feel like you've got your head around or mastered that day seems to fly out of the window and you can feel trapped, defeated and completely at the mercy of this tiny, demanding bundle.

Number one, breathe (use your Calm Breath, page 33).

Number two, there's a reason.

Number three, it doesn't last forever.

The witching hour will often begin when your baby is around two weeks old, will peak around weeks six or seven and should then start tapering off by the end of the fourth trimester. It tends to happen at around the same time every day – normally late afternoon and into the evening, say 5pm–8pm. No matter how well the day's gone, your baby seems to suddenly switch into meltdown mode, and while this

UNDERSTANDING NEWBORN STOMACH SIZES

We touched on newborn stomach sizes earlier, but during the fourth trimester at least, adapting to the aforementioned circadian rhythm is made even more difficult by a newborn's small stomach size and their subsequent need for regular food. It means sleep/awake cycles are frequent and normal, and getting your head around this will hopefully help you embrace its appropriateness and more importantly, its temporary nature. Have a look at the image below, which illustrates a newborn's stomach size during their first month of life. This really helped me to reconcile those short sleeps and frequent feeds, and hopefully it will comfort and reassure you, too.

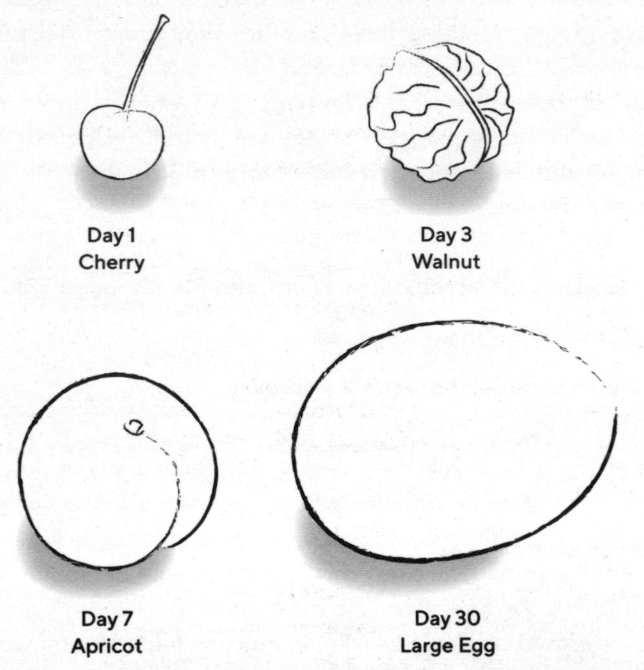

can be incredibly challenging, rest assured that it really is completely normal. As with all of these things, understanding it can ease our frustration and leave us better equipped to navigate it calmly, so let's take a closer look at what's happening.

More often than not – and the reason witching hour is so commonly linked with cluster feeding in breastfed babies – Mum's milk-making hormones (prolactin) will naturally dip at this time of day. As this happens, milk volume becomes lower and the flow slower, so baby gets frustrated at not getting what they want as quickly as they want it. This can result in them coming on and off the breast much more frequently than usual, and you thinking they're full when they're not. Offering your baby the breast frequently (even if it feels like they can't still be hungry!) is a really good idea, as not only will it support your milk supply for this time of day, but it will also help your baby to relax.

It's not just breastfed babies that experience the witching hour though, as overstimulation can also be a big factor in these fractious evenings. Think about it – the early evening is a busy time in many households; maybe older siblings are around or partners are returning from work, and there's suddenly more noise and commotion. You can often become distracted by trying to look after everyone else, your baby loses your calm and focused attention and everything starts spiralling out of control.

Since there's no hard or fast reasoning or resolution to this part of the evening, let's consider some ideas that might help us get through it with our sanity intact.

Rest on the breast

I've already touched on this one above, but offering your baby regular breastfeeds during this evening window can really help. As the volume of your milk reduces, they are likely to look for shorter, more frequent feeds than they might do during the day, so don't be afraid to follow their lead here. Even if they're not consuming loads, the act of breastfeeding helps to relax and reset your baby emotionally, especially when they're feeling fractious or unhappy. And remember that **you cannot overfeed a breastfed baby**.

Ask your household for help

If you have a partner or other children at home, ask them to be proactive, helpful and self-sufficient during this time. Perhaps your partner could prepare dinner (if you don't have a partner, this is where batch-cooking comes in super-useful, so that your evenings aren't taken up by cooking!), or entertain other children, while you are otherwise engaged. When we were in the midst of these fractious evenings with Cosmo, we'd let the bigger boys put on an episode of *Planet Earth* (or the like) and have a picnic tea in front of the television with zero guilt, because it was just about survival and keeping everyone happy. If you're on your own, a great idea is to switch your meals around so you're having a substantial warm lunch whilst baby sleeps at some point during the day, and are then able to graze or have an easy-to-prepare snack in the evening, when it's more difficult to put your baby down.

Create a calm environment

To combat overstimulation, consider small changes you can make to quieten and calm your immediate surroundings. It could be that you take your baby to a quieter room, or dim the lights and reduce any noise. This will mean your baby can feed in a more relaxed way if they are hungry, and won't be as easily distracted by household excitement and stimulation.

Wear your baby

If sitting in a quiet room isn't doable, consider wearing your baby in a sling during the witching hours. It will enable you to do other things if you need to, and your baby will feel comforted by being close to you. If you get your positioning right, it can even be possible to feed your baby while wearing them, too!

Soothing skin-to-skin

Hopefully by now you are seeing the instant soothing benefits of skin-to-skin with your baby. Skin-to-skin is something your partner could help with too, and it will really help to regulate your baby's little system and help them to relax and reset. When babies are calm, they feed more easily, so a combination of these ideas can prove effective in navigating these hairy evening hours.

Take a breather

These demanding evening sessions – however short-lived they might feel in hindsight – can be really exhausting and upsetting when you're already sleep-deprived and low on energy.

In the moments when it all feels too much, ask your partner to take over for fifteen minutes while you go and breathe, or if you're on your own, put your baby down safely and take a few moments to sit in the next room and gather your strength. You can do this. I promise.

> Sometimes the only thing we can do is take a breather, and give *ourselves* a chance to reset if we've got any hope of encouraging our baby to do the same.

COLIC

While a few hours of unsettled, fussy behaviour is very normal during these evening periods of cluster feeding or witching, some babies will seem completely inconsolable and may have prolonged periods of crying or apparent pain. This could be a sign of colic; if so then the crying will normally be paired with clenched fists, flailing arms and legs or an arched back. There is no certain cause of colic, but given that it normally begins and resolves within the fourth trimester, it's thought that it could be influenced by overstimulation (so your baby cries to release stress from sensory overload), a maturing digestive system, food sensitivity (either from something a breastfeeding mum has eaten, or an ingredient in formula), and infant reflux (again something that is naturally outgrown in most babies).

While there is no proven remedy for colic, the following ideas have lots of anecdotal support:

- Create a calm environment – as mentioned above, reducing stimulation will help your baby to relax, and this will make comforting them easier. Again, look at ways to recreate the womb – comforting your baby by recreating the security of this period will often soothe colicky babies. Dim lights, white noise, rocking your baby or wearing them in the closeness of a sling can be good ways to do this.

- Adjust baby's positioning – if stomach pain is causing your baby distress, changing the way you're holding them could help. Try the *tiger in the tree* hold (your baby lies face down, with their tummy resting on your arm) or hold them upright with their tummy against your shoulder.

- Burps and strokes – sometimes burping or releasing trapped wind will reduce the discomfort your baby is experiencing. Burping them for longer than you might normally, or incorporating some baby massage techniques, might help.

- Think about the food you're eating – it may be that your baby is reacting to something you've eaten (if you're breastfeeding) – or an ingredient in their formula. Speak to your care provider if you think this might be the case.

- Gripe water – again, there's lots of anecdotal evidence to support the efficacy of gripe water, but this will vary from baby to baby. Speak to your care provider first.

- Alternative therapies like osteopathy are really gentle and safe when you are in the experienced hands of a paediatric-trained practitioner. Osteopathy is a non-invasive hands-on therapy and is (anecdotally) very effective in calming unsettled babies by aiding the body's self-healing mechanism, which can help to restore a calmness, comfort and balance in your baby.

Remember, if your instinct is telling you that something else is going on here, don't hesitate to speak to your care providers about your concerns. Nobody knows your baby better than you, and acting on your intuition won't ever be something you regret.

CREATING CALM AMID THE CHAOS

While there's a level of joy to be found in not sweating the small stuff in these early days, I don't want to underestimate the positive effects of being able to find some peace amid the practical chaos. After all, when you're feeling tired and emotional, clutter and mess can amplify your weariness and fragility, so here are some tips to help you restore some calm in a manageable way.

1. Identify the areas at home where you'll be spending most of your time

When I was pregnant with my second son, I knew I'd be spending my immediate postnatal period in bed, and would then move to the sofa. I know that clutter does no favours for my headspace, so I acknowledged that the most important thing was that these places were calm and clean. Before my baby arrived, I took any unnecessary clutter out of these rooms (washing, piles of books, clothes/shoes that didn't need to be there etc) to make way for the inevitable extras that baby would bring, without it suddenly feeling like I had no space. Knowing that these spaces offered something of a haven meant that I could switch off to other things (dishes, laundry...) because in the short term, I didn't need to see them.

2. Create practical stations for yourself

In each of these spaces, or wherever you plan on spending those first few days/weeks, have a little bag, box or tray of the things you need on hand. For me, that was nipple cream, lip balm, a bottle/glass of water, my phone charger, a clean muslin and wipes. You could even include an affirmation card! Having these stationed where

I needed them meant I wasn't constantly on the hunt for my essentials and didn't need to cart them around the house. I know it sounds simple, but having the basics to hand can really bring about a sense of feeling calm and organised, which again resolves the conflict of other things being untidy or up in the air.

3. Prioritise the things that make you feel most at ease and ask for help with them

The reality of life with a newborn is that some jobs will inevitably fall by the wayside, but if you can identify two or three things that have the biggest impact on your headspace, you can ask your partner (or a relative/friend/doula) for help in keeping these sorted. For me, that was clean bedsheets (especially with how hot and sweaty you can get during the nights, post-partum!), fresh air and no visible clutter. If these things were sorted then I could happily turn a blind eye to an un-hoovered floor or a stack of plates in the sink! I talked to my other half about these things, and then rather than feeling overwhelmed about trying to keep the whole house in order, he could just see that these things were taken care of. I would take a bath or shower, and he would open the bedroom window, re-make the bed and put anything that didn't need to be in the bedroom in the nursery or spare room to sort later. I valued this so much, and he knew he was really helping me to feel relaxed and calm while looking after our little one. Teamwork really does make the dream work!

4. Pick one way to positively appeal to each of your senses

So here we're talking about sound, smell and sight – the easiest routes into your palpable experiences. Identify one thing that appeals to you in each of these ways, and then you can use them to transform feelings of unease or anxiety and bring about a sense of calm among any kind of chaos. Refer back to page 32, where we talked about ways to appeal effectively to your different senses.

I want to add here that chaos isn't always a tangible thing. It's not always mess, clutter and dirty washing. Sometimes chaos can be other people's opinions, conflicting advice, or a myriad answers from Dr Google. We're going to talk more about turning down this invisible noise later, but for now, know that the path to calm is via your intuition. Only when you lean in to making choices based on what feels right for you and your baby (and not what others think is right for them, or for you) does managing the maternal mental load feel less overwhelming and more like something you can take in your stride. You are learning and growing as a mother each day, and your way *is* the right way.

I am well equipped to deal with the tricky moments of motherhood

TEN TIPS FOR TINY POCKETS OF SELF-CARE

The first twelve weeks of your baby's life can feel all-consuming. When there is little sign of routine, it can be hard to know how or when to nurture yourself and keep yourself calm and sane. Try not to expect too much in terms of structure for now. It's about finding windows of opportunity for self-care and treating yourself very gently and forgivingly as you return to a more regular rhythm of life.

To personalise the idea of self-care, try to think about those things that make you feel like *you*. What did you identify with or what made you feel good pre-baby? Did you get a monthly manicure? Watch a certain TV programme? Stay on top of the news/current affairs? Identify a few appealing activities, and try to incorporate an element of them into this fourth trimester, even if it's not quite as thoroughly as you're used to!

Here are my top tips for finding tiny pockets for self-care during the all-consuming fourth trimester. Some of these may feel more achievable than others, but all of them can offer some much-needed respite from the relentless nature of the first three months. Give them a go, and don't be afraid to ask for help or support from the people around you if it will make some self-care more manageable.

- **Have a bath.** I've said it before and I'll say it again – a warm bath is an instant de-stressor and will envelop your body and calm your mind. Try using Epsom salts or essential oils for an extra element of nourishment and healing (although, as before, if you have a wound or stitches make sure you check with your midwife or care provider that this will be safe).

- **Enjoy a face mask or hair treatment.** Make the spa experience accessible with an at-home treatment – leave them on in the bath and you've got a two for one!
- **Take a walk round the block.** It's amazing what a bit of fresh air and a change of scene can do. Leave your phone at home and walk mindfully, noticing nothing more than your breathing and the sensation of your feet meeting the ground. Just go easy, and don't overdo it while your body continues to heal.
- **Listen to an audiobook or podcast.** While reading might prove a little too exhausting for your tired eyes right now, an audiobook or podcast can help give your brain a breather from the sometimes monotonous nature of these early days.
- **Eat a warm meal slowly.** I think I could count on one hand the number of hot meals/drinks I managed during the first few weeks after my babies were born, but it really is the most nourishing thing. See if someone else can hold your baby for twenty minutes while you eat with free hands. Simple pleasures!
- **Book a massage, or have your partner rub your hands or feet.** If you can afford it and have the support at home, book a massage. Having someone completely nurture and take care of you for an hour can feel so restorative and you will feel stronger and re-centred. Make sure your practitioner is qualified in postnatal massage – and some even let you take your baby with you!
- **Get a haircut or your nails painted.** Again, if set-up allows, this can be a great way of restoring a bit of energy into how you feel about yourself. Some hairdressers even offer mum/baby appointments, and you may be surprised

at how relaxing your baby finds the white noise of a hair-dryer! Lots of companies also offer at-home manicures or pedicures, which can feel like a real treat and much more accessible in the fourth trimester, when getting out of the house can sometimes feel like a logistical upheaval.

- **Read a magazine or book.** Remember when you used to do that? Next time your baby falls asleep on you, rather than reaching for your phone, pick up a magazine or book and use the opportunity of sitting down to relax and replenish your mind with something you love.
- **Take five minutes to stretch, breathe or practise some yoga.** Depending on your postnatal recovery, some gentle stretching can be a great way to re-energise the body. Pairing stretches with your breathing will help strengthen the mind–body connection, and will get those endorphins flowing too (see more on your happy hormones below).
- **Journal or draw.** There can be so much going on in our heads as we're getting used to life with our baby that it's likely to feel a bit jumbled and overwhelming at times. Writing without any pressure can be really cathartic – just see where your mind takes you and let the words flow.

HAPPY HORMONES TO THE RESCUE!

Oxytocin and endorphins are the hormones of love and help to fuse and nurture every single relationship you have. That means the relationship you have with your friends, your partner, your baby, and most importantly, yourSELF.

Our hormones have the power to make us feel certain things and experience them in different ways. When we produce adrenaline we feel tense, on edge and highly alert, whereas when we produce endorphins and oxytocin we feel happy, relaxed and at ease. While these hormones will often be produced as a reaction to what's going on around us, we can also learn to short-circuit the ones we don't need or want and trigger the production of the ones we do. If you practised hypnobirthing during your pregnancy, you'll remember the power that this simple piece of knowledge carried into your labour and birth – short-circuiting stressor hormones in order to have a more comfortable and enjoyable experience.

Something as simple as skin-to-skin with your baby, a square of your favourite chocolate, or a warm hug from a loved one can instantly get those endorphins flowing, but in this next exercise, I am going to offer up some more ideas for happy-hormone generation, and invite you to give them a go on your journey through this special time in your life.

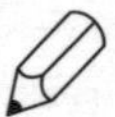

ACTIVITY

HELLO HAPPY HORMONES!

When you are tired and feeling a bit depleted, it can feel hard to identify and acknowledge feelings of comfort, happiness and love. Sometimes, though, you'll find that your mind just needs a little nudge in the right direction!

Below are five ideas I want you to try for boosting your endorphin and oxytocin production. Some will be more feasible with a newborn, and others may need to wait

until you're a little further down the line, but I want you to try to give them all a go.

Everyone will respond differently to these techniques, so I want you to give them all a mark out of ten based on how effective you felt they were. Not only will this help you to identify ways in which your personal hormonal responses work, but it will also mean you know which ones are worth revisiting when you need a happy hormone boost!

And breathe

Let's start with the most simple one – your breath! Noticing your breath and learning to regulate it can have a very profound effect on your nervous system. Whether you are standing, sitting or lying down, all I want you to do is place your awareness on the rise and fall of your breath. Relax your shoulders, soften your eyes and jaw, and now start to inhale while visualising the words 'I am safe' and exhale while visualising the words 'all is well'. Even doing this for 60 seconds can get those happy hormones fired up and flowing. If you want to practise this with even more intention, then flick back to our Heart Space Centring exercise on page 12.

Soothing strokes

Our skin is lined with nerve endings, and is such a sensitive organ. Stimulating these nerve endings can short-circuit adrenaline and prompt the production of oxytocin and endorphins, so what I want you to do is roll up one of your sleeves, and simply stroke – very gently – the inside of your arm. Work your way up from the inside of your wrist to the inside of your elbow, and try to keep this in sync with the rhythm of your breath. It has the most soothing effect and is something that can be done anytime, anywhere! This is equally a lovely one to get a partner involved in. Try it when you're watching TV or lying in bed – you'll be surprised at how instant its effects can be.

Move and be merry

Exercise and movement have an incredible impact on our endorphin levels. Now don't worry, I'm not suggesting you need to do a quick 5k to boost your happy hormones here, but finding simple ways to move your body can instantly lift your mood. In the early days and weeks with your newborn, this could include things like a good stretch, doing a few yoga sun salutations or picking three simple poses and rotating through them for five minutes, walking slowly up the stairs, and affirming something you love about yourself or are grateful for with each step, or a very slow walk around the block, inhaling peace and exhaling tension as you go. If you're longing for a chance to let loose and move your body, then put on your favourite music and have a dance around the kitchen!

Big belly laughs

We all know how amazing a good belly laugh feels, and – you guessed it – it's because laughter boosts our endorphin and oxytocin levels! Laughter also helps to alleviate physical and emotional tension, meaning that everything feels better afterwards. Those early days with your newborn can be a brilliant time to put on your all-time favourite movies and feed/snuggle your baby while you relax. If you're in need of inspiration, ask friends or your mums' group (if you have one) what the funniest movie they've ever seen is, and put that on your list for a rainy day.

Feast on your favourite foods

For most people, there are certain foods that just make us feel GOOD. That favourite meal that reminds us of our childhood, or transports us to our most treasured holiday memory. Whatever that is, cook it (or better still, get someone else to cook it for you). It's well worth getting your hands on some good-quality chocolate too, because not only will it be a nice treat to sustain all of that feeding, but it's a natural endorphin-booster!

NURTURING YOUR RELATIONSHIP WITH YOUR PARTNER

When your baby arrives, it sounds obvious to say that so much changes. But really, *so much changes*. You have a whole new person in your lives. A person whom you are wholly responsible for and who depends on you for survival. You are no longer just partners, you are parents. Your attention is divided, your resources shared, and your emotions put through the tumble dryer of love that is new parenthood!

My relationship is a safe place for love and security to flourish

During your fourth trimester (and beyond), it's completely natural for you and your partner's focus to turn towards your baby, and inevitably away from each other at times. I like to think of this as a temporary shift, because let's face it, you are both rightly in awe of this whole new human who has joined your lives. Talking to one another about what this experience is like is so important, and you should be aware that you both might be feeling differently, and that's okay too.

Try to carve out small pockets of time in these early days to check in and hold space for each other. This could be something as simple as eating breakfast or dinner together, watching an episode of your favourite show amid the evening cluster feeds, or taking baby out for a short walk in a carrier in the park and holding hands. You may both be feeling overwhelmed, but that can really be a platform to share the most wonderful empathy and intimacy with one another, and to take stock of what an amazing job you're doing as a team.

There are two things that I feel can really make a difference to your relationship in those early days with your newborn, and they are seeing and hearing each other. Really seeing and hearing each other. If you feel it would benefit you and your partner, have a go at these techniques for establishing a sense of togetherness post-birth.

I see you

One of the things a lot of couples worry about is how their physical relationship will change once they've had a baby. The reality is that your sex life may well get parked for a while, but that doesn't mean that a sense of physical togetherness needs to be lost too. Eye contact is one of the most intimate transactions we can share with another, and this exercise celebrates just that.

Set a timer for five minutes. Sit opposite your partner and hold hands. Look into each other's eyes without looking away until the timer stops. This sounds like the simplest exercise ever, I know, but it can honestly prove to be quite a wonderful challenge. You may well laugh, cry, feel horribly awkward or deeply connected – there is no right or wrong way to experience this and it may change every time you do it. What it will always bring about though, is reconnection, and that can be the most magical triumph in those early days.

I hear you

Often when we're in a relationship (of any kind), we spend lots of time talking, and even lots of time listening, but less and less time really hearing. Really hearing is about being open to another person's experience without trying to influence it with our own. It's actually a really hard thing to do, because often our natural default is to try to empathise and make things better for someone. When someone tells us they're finding something really hard, we can hear that as a call for us to try to make it better, and the acknowledgment of it being hard, and what that feels like, can get lost.

In this exercise, I invite you and your partner to hear each other. Set aside a small pocket of time to ask each other how they are feeling, and challenge yourself to say nothing when the other person speaks. If one of you is feeling particularly exhausted or short-tempered, that is just to be heard and not be met with any type of defence, reaction or solution. Again, this can be a hugely intimate exercise, because it's offering the ultimate gift of a safe space being held for you, without any judgement or expectation. And again, the more you do it, the easier it gets – you'll see that for yourselves, I promise.

ACTIVITY

KINDNESS JAR

It's natural for the romance in your relationship to be replaced with a different type of love during your fourth trimester, but that doesn't mean love, intimacy and kindness can't flourish between you during this time – it might just look a bit different.

When we're tired and emotional, we can often stop seeing and feeling the love and care present in our relationship so readily. This exercise offers a simple opportunity to appreciate and value each other, whenever you need it most.

1. **Get a few sheets of paper, ideally in two different colours.**
2. **Write kind statements or things you appreciate about your partner on one of the pieces of coloured paper. Cut each one out and fold it up.**

3. Ask your partner to do the same on the other-colour paper.
4. Pop all of the pieces of paper into a jar – let's say green paper is notes for you, and red is notes for your partner. When either of you are feeling a bit low or unappreciated, dip into the kindness jar and read a loving statement from your partner. It works a treat and will always be on hand when you need it most.

Keep topping up your jar as the days and weeks go by. If your partner does something kind or that you appreciate – however small – jot it down and pop it in the jar. Encourage them to do the same so that the jar retains a balance of each colour.

TWO WEEKS LATER

If you have a partner and they've been able to take parental leave, it's likely that they'll be returning to work a couple of weeks after your baby's been born, or maybe earlier. Perhaps you're a family who have decided to take shared parental leave. Whatever your plans, this can be a huge transition for you both, as it can feel, in a way, that this special bubble that you've been living in has involuntarily burst. Of course, it can be an invaluable practical help to have an extra pair of hands on deck to share the logistics of life with your new baby, but there's also the emotional landscape that can be easier to navigate when the person you love is close by. Having another adult in the house to offer practical help and emotional reassurance is of such value, and I think it's a good idea to talk about this transition together and acknowledge that it's likely to be difficult for you both when a normal(ish) routine resumes.

Let's think about how we can make this back-to-work transition an easier one, and give you some coping and calming strategies for when you're at home on your own with baby.

CHECK-IN TIME

While a work day might fly by (especially when you're looking forward to getting home and seeing baby), it can sometimes feel like the hours are crawling for the person who's at home with baby. Get your partner to set an alarm (or two) in their phone so they can just send you a text or give a quick call to check in with you. Having those little landmarks through the day where you know your partner is thinking of you can be a real help in the early days.

EXTENDED NETWORKS

Let your extended network know when your partner is returning to work, so that they can offer extra support where needed. If you've maintained an intimate baby bubble for the first couple of weeks of your baby's life, now can be a nice time to start introducing your baby to some close friends and family. Saving this for week two or three means that you have something to look forward to by way of company, without it compromising the sacred time for you and your partner. Now would be a good time to revisit our ideas around asking for what you need on pages 30 and 3.

REACH OUT

In a time where your baby's needs are still so full-on and their routine unpredictable, it might not always be easy to make actual plans with people, but remember that you can still reach out when you need to. Text your partner or call a friend if you're having a hard day or need to vent – these feelings are always more manageable when we share them, and even a kind word back can give us the reassurance and comfort we need.

HOME TIME

The most eagerly awaited part of your day, especially in these early days, will be the return of adult company and someone to share your baby's demands with. Talk about what your home-time routine will look like so that you're both on the same page. Maybe you could agree that when your partner gets home from work, they could give your baby a bath or wear them in the sling for half an hour while you get into a warm bath. It will give you both a little dose of what you've been missing, and it offers a welcome breather at the end of those long days.

NURTURING YOUR NEWEST LOVE

Bonding is a hot topic among new parents, but I think it's good to keep in mind that there isn't a one-size-fits-all approach when it comes to nurturing loving bonds. I also think it's important to remember that these new connections aren't only between you and your baby. Bringing a baby into the world is likely to have a profound impact on your relationship, friendships, familial relations and even your place in the professional world; but for now let's focus on your little one.

When we talk about bonding, we often think about an intense feeling of love that should appear as soon as our baby does, but actually, the pace and growth of bonding is unique to each parent. Rather than put ourselves under the pressure of what we believe love or bonding *should* look like, I think it's healthier to explore how we can create the space and environment in which this love can deepen and grow as you get to know your baby. This will have the biggest impact on how your attachment relationships build over time, and I talk about this idea of ongoing bonding in more detail on pages 159 and 257.

In terms of developing nurturing bonds with your baby, we talked about the benefits of skin-to-skin, talking to your baby, singing songs or reading books and mirroring your baby's expressions and movements back on page 24. These all offer such simple and effective ways to really connect with your baby on a level they can subconsciously engage with, and I would really encourage you to incorporate them all on a daily basis during the fourth trimester and beyond.

When I work with expectant mums, I often talk about bonding as *closeness,* and you can refresh your memory on the importance of this if you head back to the section on meeting the needs of your baby (see page 45). I think we can subconsciously attach a lot of pressure to the word bonding, whereas closeness feels more within our reach without overthinking. Essentially, closeness can be the most valuable thing to provide for your baby in those early weeks and months, and when we think about it from a physiological perspective, it makes sense.

As we had an opportunity to think about with the Making Womb exercise (see page 46), while your baby grows inside your tummy, they become used to hearing your voice and the voices of those close to you frequently. This becomes a reassuring sound for your baby, so it's easy to understand why they want to remain so close to you once they've transitioned into the world. Your heartbeat has also been a constant comfort for them, which is why they're always likely to be settled and sleep soundly with their head on your chest. Be mindful of this when you bring your baby home and start introducing them to the other people in their lives. YOU are their safe place, and if they seem fractious when they're apart from you, it's only because they are still getting used to things here. Frequent contact and lots of skin-to-skin will help your baby realise that they are safe and secure, and from there, their relationships with others have the platform to thrive.

Remember that you and your partner will find your own special ways to bond with your baby, and it's normal for this to deepen and develop at different paces. Try talking to friends who've had babies and ask them what their favourite ways to bond were. You may have found more of your own special ways to bond, too. Write them down here so that you can look back on them fondly and remember how you spent the early days getting to know each other. This is one of those logs that you'll be so glad you made a year from now.

ACTIVITY

HERE'S LOOKING AT YOU, BABY

One of the simplest and most effective ways to bond and connect with your baby is through touch and eye contact. Your newborn baby can only see about 20 to 40 centimetres ahead of them – basically enough to make out the person offering them closeness and care, which is very likely to be you right now!

In this activity – and this is one that can be enjoyed anytime and anywhere – I want you to simply mirror your baby's facial movements and expressions. Many of us have this idea that babies are pretty boring and do very little during their first few weeks and months, but actually, if you give a baby's face your undivided attention for five minutes, you'll notice quite the opposite! They are actively trying to process and make sense of so many things, and this often requires a lot of comfort and reassurance on your part, because the world can be a scary place when everything's so new.

By holding your baby close, enjoying eye contact, and mirroring their expressions, you are showing that you are watching and listening, and this helps to build secure attachment bonds between you. We often try to stimulate our baby with toys or sounds that promise endless entertainment, but actually, moments of your undivided attention and emotional availability are far more valuable in the long term.

Use the space here to jot down what you notice each time you try this with your baby. Do they scrunch their face up? Do they sneeze, yawn, even smile? Does their breathing slow down or speed up? Are they making any noises? Keeping an ongoing log of this will really help you to become more in tune with their ways of communicating, and strengthen that wonderful, growing bond.

HELPING YOUR OTHER CHILDREN ADAPT TO A NEW ARRIVAL

If you already have children, there are lots of ways that you can help them adapt to having a new baby in the house. In my experience, it's something women can feel very anxious about ahead of their little one's arrival, but with a bit of forward planning and empathy, it can be a really exciting and joyful time in your family.

Hopefully you've talked to your other child(ren) lots during your pregnancy about what life might look like when baby arrives, but here are some ideas to help you nurture these new relationships and keep the transition as stress-free as possible, especially during the fourth trimester.

A lot will depend on the age of your child or children. Very young children may seem upset, confused or clingy when their baby brother or sister arrives, whereas older ones may be more excited and keen to be involved. Take things at your child's pace, and be open to hearing their experience, even if it isn't as you'd envisaged. This will go a long way in helping them to feel secure and supported in the trickier bits of this journey too.

INCORPORATING OTHER CHILDREN INTO YOUR FOURTH TRIMESTER

Toddlers (let's say one- to three-year-olds)

It's unlikely that the really little ones will understand what all of this means, and more than anything will probably be looking for reassurance and love. Skin-to-skin is the wonder hormone for everyone and letting your toddler cosy up with you and baby will be calming and emotionally beneficial to you all. Even cosying up together after bath time to read a book or have a cuddle will initiate these feelings of closeness and togetherness.

Pre-schoolers (so three- to five-year-olds)

For children who are old enough to understand the concept of a new baby a little more, jealousy can present more strongly. Obviously, when you're feeling tired and fragile yourself this can affect you more profoundly, so it's a good thing to be mindful of and it's important to remind yourself that it's completely normal. It can be a really great idea to talk to your pre-schooler about what you're doing when you're looking after your baby. You could get them a special doll or soft animal that they can take care of alongside you, so that they feel involved and part of your team.

Another nice idea is to have them draw pictures or create some art for the new baby. Not only will the creativity help them to express what they're feeling, but it's a nice opportunity for them to feel valuable and celebrated. When you're feeding your baby (especially the late afternoon/evening cluster feeds in those first few months!), your bigger little one could snuggle up with you and watch some TV – this will probably feel like a treat for them and they can enjoy that closeness with you too.

Older children

Children aged five plus may also present feelings of jealousy alongside the excitement of having a new sibling. Again, creating artwork is a brilliant outlet for their emotions, and a precious gift for baby too. It can also be a valuable activity to make a little list with them about all the good things about being older. Maybe it's eating tastier foods, staying up later, getting to dress up or play games with their friends. Focusing on the positives while offering your emotional availability to hold space for the trickier bits will make everyone's transition into your new family dynamic a happier one.

TOP TIPS FOR A HARMONIOUS HOMECOMING

- Encourage siblings to create a piece of art for the new baby (or have a go at making those Presence Pebbles on page 60 together) – this is such a brilliant way to help children of all ages express themselves and have an opportunity to celebrate their feelings.
- Give each child individual attention when possible – this could be something as simple as helping them get dressed or brush their hair, or having a game of snap while baby sleeps.
- Include older siblings in photos – your child is probably used to being the centre of attention, and while you'll be snapping away at your newest addition, make sure you're still capturing lots of your other child too, or even invite them to be photographer!
- Involve older children – think of age-appropriate ways for older children to feel involved in caring for their baby sibling rather than put-upon. Maybe they could sing to baby, pass you wipes or nappies, help rub baby's back after a feed, or help to make you comfy. Let them know that you appreciate it when they are kind, helpful, loving or caring; it will make them feel proud and remind them that they have an important and valuable place in your family.
- Baby brings a present – this seems to be a really popular one, and successful too. If there's something your older child has been coveting for a while, getting baby to 'bring it home' for them can score instant popularity points!
- Praise good behaviour – it sounds obvious but it can be easy to feel on edge and protective when you bring your baby

home, so make sure you focus on praising your older child's good behaviour. This is likely to encourage more of the same.

- Talk and hear – it's important to remember that how you envisage or expect your child to feel might not line up with their reality. Be open to hearing how they really feel and offer them a safe space to talk to you without feeling judged or reprimanded. It's normal for other children to feel angry, sad or jealous to start with, and having a safe space to explore this with you will make difficult feelings easier to process.

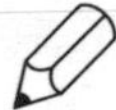

ACTIVITY

LOVE NOTES TO YOUR LITTLE ONE

This is a really simple activity that can be tailored in an age-appropriate way depending on the age of your other children. It also works well during a time where you are likely to be spending a lot of time sitting/lying with your baby for hours at a time. The fourth trimester can often bring the most intense time of struggle for older siblings because of its consuming nature, so this simple activity can prove a big help.

Your notes don't have to be long or time-consuming, just little notes reminding them how well they're doing and how much you love them. Invite them to write back to you, and maybe have a secret place where you leave these notes for each other in exchange. This

helps to make it feel precious and like something that is just about you two, and can go a really long way in reassuring other children of how loved they are.

Your notes could include things like:

> *'I was so proud of you today when you got your shoes on all by yourself. You're so smart!'*
>
> *'Seeing you become a big brother/sister really amazes me – you are doing such a brilliant job.'*
>
> *'When you sang today, baby stopped crying – they must love the sound of your voice and I do too.'*

Depending on the age of your child, when they 'write back' to you, they may include things that they're feeling anxious or worried about, but don't want to say out loud. Writing to each other can offer a brilliant safe space for this, and you can show that you hear and value their experience in your replies.

My home is safe
and full of love

A FINAL THOUGHT

If you digest one idea about you and your baby's fourth trimester, let it be that it is completely normal for these first few weeks and months to feel like an absolute whirlwind. Your baby's adjustment to being born is just as huge and profound as yours as a mother, and this time is about getting to know each other, and easing in to this new and beautiful relationship. It's likely you'll feel that there is no rhyme and reason to anything your baby is doing right now – no glimpse of a routine, no 'norm' and no predictability – but the key to finding joy in that is to celebrate its sacred and short-lived nature. There is so much more to come, but right now, all your baby needs is you. Surrendering to the unknown, soaking up those sweet newborn smells and cuddles, and treating yourself as softly and kindly as you do them, will mean you can cherish these first moments together and thrive into motherhood, your way.

SPACE TO REFLECT

SPACE TO REFLECT

PART THREE

RESURFACING: A NEW REALITY (3–6 MONTHS)

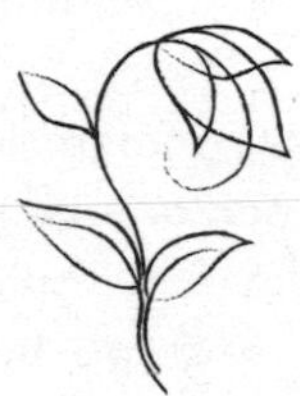

RELAX AND RESURFACE

The first twelve weeks of your baby's life have a peculiar way of feeling like a lifetime and the blink of an eye, all in one go. At moments, time seems to stand still and you feel as if you'll forever be held captive by this tiny little milk monster. There will have been long days of holding, carrying, rocking, feeding, shushing, patting and singing. Days where you've had no adult conversation and days where you have no idea what time it is. There will have been days that you've felt like crying, and days where you've felt overwhelmed with love and pride for this little baby who adores you. Days you've wanted to run away and days you can't imagine having wanted to be anywhere else. There will have been days that felt like they'd never end, and weeks that flashed by in a heartbeat. Such are the sleep-deprived, love-fuelled, often disorientating demands of the fourth trimester.

Now that your baby is three months old (or thereabouts), there are likely to be small shifts afoot. Your baby is starting to adapt to life outside of the womb, and you are becoming adept and more confident in meeting their needs and responding to the nuances of their calls (see page 152 for more on this). Take a moment to recognise that. You are doing so well. You have been doing the most relentless work for the last twelve weeks and it's time to start reaping and recognising your rewards. You are your baby's whole world – you have made them feel safe, secure and unconditionally loved, and as you don't get many appraisals in this motherhood game, I want to take a moment to tell you just how ***well*** you have done. Seriously. You deserve a pay rise.

Around this time is often when women start feeling like they want to start reconnecting with the world around them. Try not to think about going backward or forward here, but rather *rejoining*, and know that you're exactly where you're meant to be. If you have felt this way sooner, that's normal, and similarly, if you want to hang out in your bubble a little longer, that's fine too! Hopefully you will be noticing that your intuition on these things is serving you well, and that your way *is* the right way here. There is no *wrong*.

In this section, we're going to be looking at how you might be feeling as you settle into motherhood, and I'm going to be encouraging you more than ever to believe in yourself and embrace finding your own way. We're going to explore how you might be feeling about your identity, your body, your intuition, and getting a clearer sense of what motherhood *your way* looks like. We're also going to be acknowledging and understanding what's going on for your baby, and how you can continue to support and nurture their development in a mindful, centred and loving way. We'll talk about connecting with those around you, and finding your tribe who will become a network of empathy, encouragement and enjoyment for you and your baby, whatever your set-up. And then, of course, I'll be sharing some practical tips and simple exercises to help you get the most out of your experiences along the way.

The transition between zero to three and three to six months can feel like a pretty significant one. While you may well feel excited at your growing confidence and your baby's emerging personality, it's easy to start piling on the comparisons with those around you, too. To kick things off in this new step on your journey, I want to share with you a really brilliant anchoring technique that will help to re-centre your thoughts, allow you to reconnect with your confidence, and calm any stresses when life starts to feel overwhelming.

ACTIVITY

TAKE FIVE

The Take Five technique uses your five digits to draw on your own subconsciously logged memories of enjoyable, relaxing and strength-affirming experiences. By connecting with times when we've felt happy, capable and at ease, we can bring forward the emotions associated with those into our current space. It's really easy to do anywhere and at any time, and the more you do it, the more adept you'll become at generating good feelings and drawing on their power and strength when you need it most.

Here's how to do it, and you can use the illustration overleaf to write down a positive memory on each finger, so that you always have it to look back on and refer to.

1. Touch your thumb to your index finger. As you do, take your mind back to a time when your body felt physically strong and healthy, and where you experienced that post-activity endorphin high. Maybe you completed a run, swim, or maybe it was the feeling you had after you gave birth!
2. Next, touch your thumb to your middle finger. As you do, take your mind back to a time when you had a loving experience. This could be anything from an intimate conversation to an amazing hug or sexual experience. Feel the warmth and connectedness of that moment again now.
3. Touch your thumb to your ring finger. As you do, take your mind back to the nicest compliment you have ever received. Who gave it to you and what did they say? How did it make you feel in that moment? Try to really appreciate that lovely compliment now.
4. Touch your thumb to your little finger. As you do, take your mind back to the most peaceful or beautiful place you have ever visited. This could be a holiday or a place from your childhood – anywhere that feels happy and loving for you. Try to connect with what it looks, sounds and smells like and really transport yourself there in your mind's eye.

The Take Five exercise is at your fingertips, takes less than five minutes and is incredibly effective in generating a renewed sense of confidence, calmness

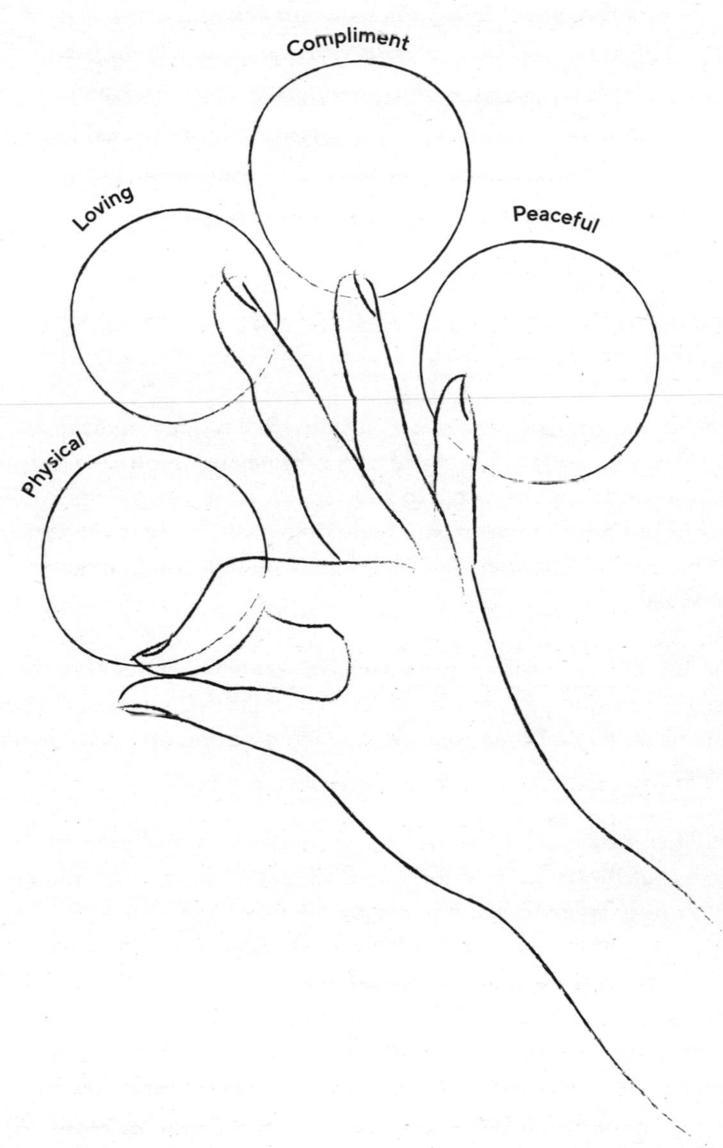
Compliment
Loving
Peaceful
Physical

and relaxation. Trying it in moments of stress or tension will mean you learn to short-circuit your body's stressor responses, and generate the production of the hormones that make you feel stronger, safer and more peaceful. It's an amazing exercise for mums, and even better when you can teach it to your little ones, too!

RECOGNISING YOUR WORTH AND REFRAMING PRODUCTIVITY

One of the trickier things about this time is that life begins to move quickly again and the novelty of a squishy newborn (and the support of their fan base) can begin to subside. Whether people are cooing over your little one or not, you remain the one meeting your baby's needs, and doing the majority of this invisible and undervalued workload.

Because our productivity as mothers isn't particularly measurable (or visible), it can sometimes lead to feelings of inadequacy, but I'm here to remind you that your work is absolutely amazing and actually, life-changing.

Yes, it can still sometimes feel horribly relentless and exhausting at times, but giving yourself the love and credit you deserve will go a long way in spurring you on to enjoy this ride, your way.

It is easy to think of motherhood as a concept that spans time and generations, but actually, our experience of motherhood is dramatically affected by the time, society and culture that we are living in. Think about it. Many years ago, women had children much younger and were often unlikely to have had a career beforehand, or would have been ready to give it up for good when their baby arrived. Their path *was* motherhood (often whether they liked it or not, I'd imagine) and while this would have brought with it its own pressures and strains, it was nonetheless considered 'enough' of a full-time occupation. There's a lot to be said for that.

Like many working mothers, I often imagine how I'd feel – or how differently I'd feel – about motherhood if I felt nothing *else* was expected of me. How would I feel if my day's work – looking after my child – was considered completely enough by the society around me: if keeping them fed, warm, loved and happy was of such value that it *understandably* took up all of my time, resources and headspace? Having seen my own mother – an incredible stay-at-home mum to my brother and me – struggle emotionally when we grew up and left home, I know that a big part of me feels relieved that I can nurture and celebrate other parts of my identity and skills, but I'm all too aware that with that comes its own pressure. Being a full-time mother is absolutely and completely a full-time job, and only when we start identifying it as such can we really acknowledge how well we are doing, even when it doesn't feel that way. I think it's fair to say that this is one of the most-talked about conflicts of modern motherhood.

We only have to reflect on how we feel when we're asked what we do by well-meaning others if our answer is 'mother', or as it always comes out: 'I'm just a mum'. *Just* a mum. Just a mum? No matter how ridiculous it seems for us to say that, we fall into the trap, immediately writing off any acknowledgement for the physical and emotional hard work we're unconditionally completing, day in, day out. The work that gets no pay, no lunch break, no sick days, holidays or a Christmas party. It's of little surprise that doing something that gets such little tangible recognition or remuneration leaves us feeling like our efforts barely justify being identified as work, and as such, it's vital that we learn to recognise and value our own worth and productivity in other ways.

While this mental reframing of our worth is unlikely to happen overnight, I really want to invite you to start acknowledging the work you're doing as valuable, profound and hugely beneficial not only to your child, but to the society you're contributing to.

I truly believe that mothers are capable of having the biggest impact on a wider world. After all, it is the little people we are raising and loving who will lead on.

How we nurture and parent our children will have profound effects on the adults they become and their contributions to humankind. I think work rarely gets more badass (or important!) than that.

I am a good mother

ACTIVITY

A MAMA'S WORTH

How many times have you heard a friend say that she appreciated her own mother more on becoming a mother herself? I know that was certainly true for me, and I think it's a feeling that many new mothers can relate to. Even if your maternal relationships aren't straightforward, I'm confident that when you're in it yourself you get a newfound respect for the hard work and unconditional love that's involved.

Sadly, this is not always the belief that our cultural narrative would have us believe. So much of our society is valued by economic input, and when women step out of the workforce (permanently, temporarily or flexibly) the value of their work is subconsciously downgraded. We can all be, at times, guilty of compliance in this social narrative, so I think it's really important that we actively acknowledge the worth of a mother, for ourselves if no one else.

In this activity, I'm inviting you to identify the work and contribution of a mother. Use the empty heart overleaf to write down the assets, skills and contributions that a mother makes for her children and society. Consider all of the things you are (or will be) helping your child

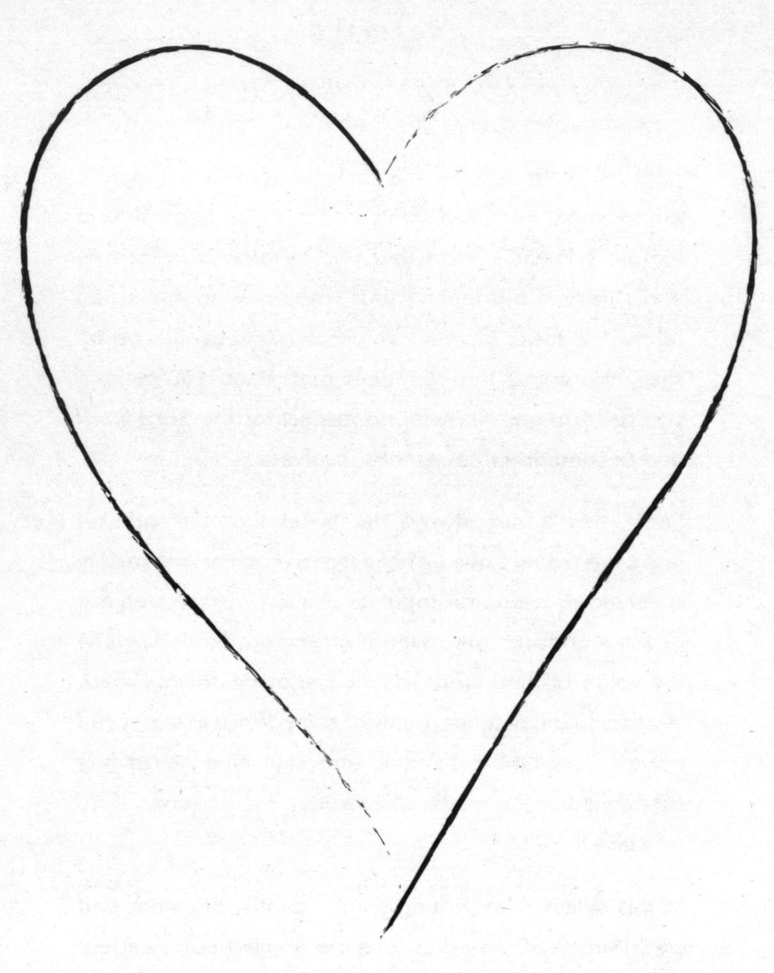

to learn and navigate over the coming years, and how your work is shaping the person they will become.

Maybe you'll include things like modelling empathy, offering comfort, unconditional loving, feeding, exploring nature, teaching language – there is so much scope, but I want to encourage you to go about this your own way. Identifying these contributions from your own perspective will also help you to tune in to the calling of your own instincts and beliefs, and we want *this* to lead the way in your onward journey.

Filling up this heart with the value and output of a mother will help you to identify your worth and reframe your productivity when it doesn't manifest in such a traditional way.

I do not need to compare myself to other people

WHAT'S HAPPENING, BABY?

We've already explored the general consensus that there is no rhyme or reason to most things that happen in your baby's first twelve weeks on Earth. Their sleep is all over the place – lots of snoozing in the day and feeding at night – they are happiest when held, and their mood/appetite can prove unpredictable at best in those early days. When this is what we expect, we can get to grips with its up-and-down nature, but I think it can be healthy to apply some of this approach on our forward journey, too. After all, it's not as if at twelve weeks your baby realises the fourth trimester is over and suddenly revises their schedule to do things 'by the book'.

Just like due dates, this is another thing your baby has no concept of, and as such, each baby's development will be slightly different. While all babies will go through physical and cognitive leaps, there remains a lot of movement around the readiness of each baby in reaching these. Remember that you and your baby are completely unique, and that is something to embrace, rather than obsess over. That said, a baby who is three to six months old will normally start offering up more predictability over feeding and sleeping, and if we learn to recognise these natural structures, we can gently nurture them and finally feel like we are falling into a more relaxed rhythm of motherhood.

FOR THE LOVE OF SLEEP

Remember this though: All babies are good. Even the ones who don't sleep. **There is no such thing as a bad baby.** Babies often won't sleep consistently or predictably during their first year, and this doesn't make them bad. They're not lying or stealing things or littering, they're just sleeping like babies sleep – sporadically and in a way their changing needs demand. Now that's not to say that we all wouldn't value more of those glorious zzzs, but I think it's healthier to consider ways we can gently nurture better relationships with sleep, rather than get ourselves tangled up in this obsession for it to be a certain way at a certain point.

We've already talked about their slow adaptation to the circadian rhythm during the fourth trimester (see page 100), but now that your baby is around the three-to-six-month mark, you may notice that your days start presenting some more predictable patterns as they become better acquainted with it. That doesn't mean that every day is going to be the same, but you may start to feel more attuned to your baby's norms, and that's because you're always learning more about each other, too. Their activity will tend to follow some kind of food/play/sleep rhythm, and it's likely that a decent morning nap will start becoming a steady feature of their day. Whereas the first twelve weeks are pretty much eat/sleep-based, you'll notice that there's more awake time now too, and this is because your baby is starting to learn, observe and adapt to the world around them – working hard to acquire the new tools that will support their ongoing development.

We can use our deeper understanding of our baby's cues and patterns to our advantage. Whether that's knowing when we're more able to bag a nap for ourselves, plan a car journey or schedule in some journaling, cleaning, organising or self-care, becoming more familiar with our baby's loose patterns of activity can offer up glimpses for the calmness and control you can slowly return to, if you so wish.

Because every baby will navigate this differently, 'how-to' books and manuals can seem overwhelming and even discouraging. Try, instead, to follow your baby's own unique cues and signals for what they want when. Since the day they were born, they have been communicating with you in their own way, and over the last few months you have been learning this new language together.

On the days that you're doubting yourself, take a moment to remind yourself that you've completely met your baby's needs every single day and recognise how amazing that is.

You are learning so much, and just because things don't always go to plan, it doesn't mean you're not doing a brilliant job at navigating and adapting to your baby's needs.

ACTIVITY

ACTIVE, STILL, FUSSY

A really good way to identify your baby's sleep readiness is to think about his/her awake time in three stages – active, still and fussy. An active baby will be watching you and what is happening around them and they may appear engaged and ready to interact. They will be responsive to your facial expressions and will try to communicate with you through sounds and movement. They seem happy to be awake. Because babies' brains are so small and the world offers so much stimulation, it's natural that they get tired quickly at this young age.

After an active period, it's likely that your baby will become still, and this signifies that they are beginning

to feel tired and may be ready to sleep. A still baby may be quieter, not seem so engaged in what you're doing, or stare off at things. Although they may not be rubbing their eyes or yawning (cues we generally associate with tiredness), this is the ideal time to encourage sleep.

Beyond the still stage comes fussiness, and this is when babies have become overtired. It's a bit like us getting ratty and short-tempered when we're running on empty, and you may notice them rubbing their eyes, making agitated sounds, or generally not being happy with any interaction from you.

A great way to start strengthening your understanding of your baby on a deeper and more personal level is to keep a little journal of *their* norms. What are *their* active signs, what are *their* still signs and what are *their* fussy signs? It's all very well reading templates and guidelines for age-appropriate sleep, but it's being able to recognise the individual nuances in *your* baby that will enhance your intuition over these things and make speaking (and hearing) their language so much easier.

In the illustration overleaf, there are three sleep clouds labelled Active, Still and Fussy. In each cloud, jot down some words or behaviours that capture what your baby is like in each of these stages. Getting a sense of which characteristics fall into which stage of their awake time will help you to recognise their still stage more

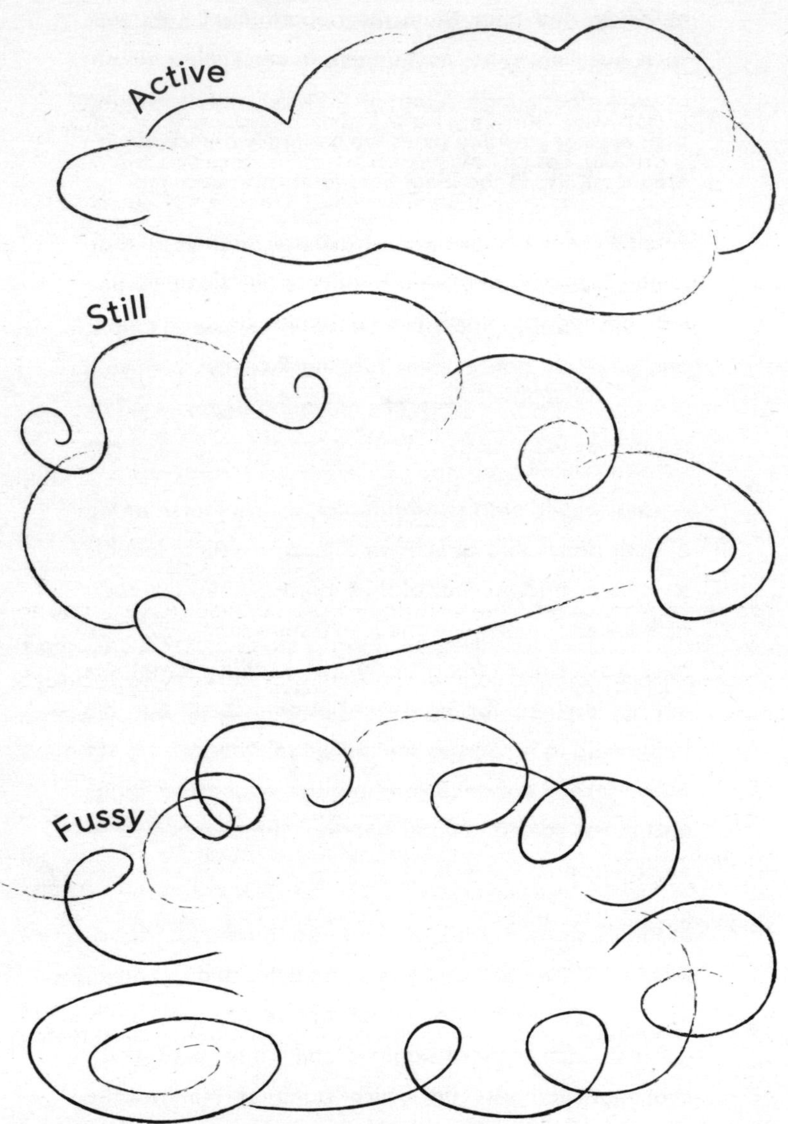
Active
Still
Fussy

intuitively, and offer them the opportunity of a sleep when it is likely to be most beneficial and well received.

To start with, you may have trouble deciphering which stage your baby is in, but once you've observed them for a few days with this in mind, I bet you'll begin identifying them more easily, and this can be a real game-changer in gently nurturing positive sleep habits, and boosting your confidence and intuition too.

It's very normal to feel overwhelmed when you're trying to work out what your baby wants from you – what their different sounds mean or how to meet their needs in ever-changing ways, but observation really is one of the best ways to become more familiar and confident in learning about your baby. You'll be amazed at how much you can learn from quiet observations, so I'd really encourage you to do this actively from time to time. It can be as simple as keeping a notebook to hand, and jotting down the hallmarks of your baby's behaviour at different times of day. For example, do they rub their face and eyes a lot around a certain time? Prefer lying down or being upright at others? Seem happier being held by someone else after a feed but only want you when they wake up? These signs and signals can seem insignificant on their own, but think of them as pieces of a puzzle that are much more substantial and informative when gathered together.

LET'S PLAY!

As your baby moves forward through their fourth trimester and into the three-to-six-month period, you will begin to get a sense that they are becoming much more familiar with their environment and the people in it. Their eating and sleeping habits are starting to become more settled, and they are starting to connect with the idea of play. While you may think there isn't much your baby will be able to do yet, you'll soon learn that they respond to the simplest of things being fun, and this can offer some brilliant opportunities to deepen your bond and connect intuitively and lovingly.

At this stage in their emotional development, your baby is also becoming more discriminate in their attachment relationships. Rather than being quite so happy to have their needs met by anyone available, you may notice that they are specifically looking for, and more easily comforted by you, above others. Incorporating play into the time you spend with your baby can really help to solidify this sense of security, whilst creating some wonderful opportunities for you to learn about their developing personality and their likes and dislikes. You may start getting really positive or animated reactions around certain activities, and you can log this as something your baby loves. Similarly, there may be things that your baby just isn't interested in, and this can inform how you nurture and play with them, too.

Play is such an important part of childhood, and even though your baby is still tiny, this is an incredible gateway to deeper connection, learning and communication. Enjoy these moments with your baby, and carve out pockets of time where you can put distractions aside and really tune in to who this little person is, and who you are too.

ACTIVITY

FIRST GLIMPSES OF FUN

A lot of the play at this young age will be a continuation of the bonding activities we looked at earlier in the book – eye contact, skin-to-skin and talking/singing to baby (see pages 24–26) – but here are some other simple ideas for building on these lovely moments of connection to teach your baby about play. Remember to keep things simple, don't put too many expectations on their reactions or the 'success' of playing, and focus instead on the little moments of intimacy and happiness that can be found among these playful interactions.

Use the space overleaf to note down how your baby reacts to these games, as it will give you a good idea of the activities they find enjoyable and stimulating, and will serve as a lovely record to look back on. You could even print some photos of their first reactions to play and keep them here as a memento of those little firsts.

Rub a dub dub

Give your baby a massage. Use some gentle oil that you've warmed in your hands, and try incorporating a nursery rhyme or song that involves round-and-round movements.

Peek-a-boo

This is a firm favourite for babies of all ages, but remember to start gently. You could use a muslin or small piece of coloured cloth to hide and reappear from.

Nursery rhymes

The sing-song, simple nature of nursery rhymes makes them super-appealing to baby's early senses. It's never too early to introduce your baby to storytelling, and remember that their future verbal skills are built upon the hours they spend hearing your soothing, familiar voice.

Nature watch

If the weather is nice, lie outside on a blanket and enjoy the sensory offerings of nature. You may see trees blowing in the breeze, clouds moving, or birds chirping and flying. The benefits of vitamin D and exposure to sunlight will also mean that their melatonin levels are boosted, and as this is our sleep hormone, it could have other positive effects at home too!

Mirror Mirror

A lovely way to encourage tummy-time for little ones is to have a few strategically placed mirrors for them to discover. Imagine spotting yourself for the first time and how fun that would be! They can also be good fun in the bath or in different lighting.

LEARNING TO LOVE AND RECONNECT WITH YOUR BODY

Since becoming a mother, I genuinely believe that the body of a woman is one of the greatest and most intricate celebrations of love. What our bodies do in our reproductive years is nothing short of miraculous, and so often this is unrecognised or worse, berated. In our capitalist, western culture, we are not in the habit of loving and appreciating the uniqueness and changing nature of our bodies. In fact, quite the opposite is true. We are bombarded with the idea that attractiveness is slim, toned, tanned and so on, and then when we become mothers these messages are ramped up to include 'bouncing back', 'ditching the mum tum', 'yummy mummy' and 'getting our body back'. Mama, your body hasn't gone anywhere. It's been with you this whole time – growing, stretching, birthing, feeding, comforting, holding, squeezing. It's been working. It's been working and loving and nurturing hard, and while 'loving your body' might still feel like a way off right now, we can certainly start showing it some of the kindness it deserves, and has well and truly earned.

Challenges aside, most women will have experienced a newfound respect and admiration for their bodies at some point during their pregnancy. The beautiful bump that houses our baby, bigger boobs for those of us who aren't normally used to them, glowing skin and luscious locks feel easy to celebrate, and we often hear from others that we're blooming. But fast-forward nine months, and how many people say that to a new mum? I don't think I've ever heard it, that's for sure. It's more likely that we'll be told we look tired or that we've got sick on our shoulder, and that fall from grace in less than a year can feel pretty harsh (and have an obvious impact on our self-esteem).

What I'm inviting you to do is to see your body – 'flaws' and all – as living proof of your journey to date. Every time you look in the mirror and see the changed bits staring back at you – especially the ones you may consider less appealing like eye bags or stretch marks – I want you to focus on the story behind them. So instead of 'my eyes look tired', try 'my eyes look tired because I was up all night feeding and cuddling my gorgeous baby', or instead of 'I hate my stretch marks', try 'my stretch marks are a precious memento of all the growing and nurturing my body has done'. Changing our internal dialogue can really help to piece together the disconnect between the reality we feel and the reality we're sold, and that, Mama, is the enlightenment that every woman deserves.

A big part of this reconnection is about finding joy in our bodies again. We've already talked a lot about rest and nourishment (see tips for self-care on page 113), but there is space for pleasure, enjoyment and celebration of ourselves again, too. Take time to reflect on your fond memories involving your body – anything from swimming in the sea, to amazing sex, to a physical achievement you trained for – this is about reconnecting with the strength and capabilities of your body and its ever-changing nature.

When we proactively create shifts in our internal dialogue, we make way for finding this joy in our bodies again. Whether this is through exercise, dancing, fashion or physical pleasure, there is so much opportunity to reconnect with our evolving bodies and find ourselves right there where we always were. These things might feel physically or emotionally different to how they once used to, and going gently with yourself is most certainly the key, but know that this isn't the end of your physical self – it's a whole new beginning, and one that goes *your way*.

The one thing I've learned from watching my body change/grow/birth/nurture over the last ten years is that body love and kindness has got to start from within. That the most important and valuable source of appreciation comes from ourselves, and that the more loving we feel towards our bodies, the more confidently we can celebrate them. In this next exercise, I'm going to be inviting you to celebrate the new and changed parts of you – the softness of your exterior and the strength of your insides. It may feel difficult or even uncomfortable to try this at first, but I promise that the more you try it, the easier it will become.

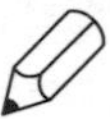

ACTIVITY

A WEEK OF COMPLIMENTS

On the next page, you'll see that there are seven boxes, labelled Monday to Sunday. Every day, when you wake up, I want you to stand in front of the mirror and look at your reflection. This may feel uncomfortable at first, but try to breathe, relax your shoulders and know that you are safe. I want you to look into your own eyes and say, either out loud or in your mind, 'I see you', and then I want you to give yourself a compliment.

If this feels like a difficult thing to do, then imagine when you're looking in the mirror that you are looking at a friend. Study her, give her hand a squeeze and immerse yourself in her energy, and then say the loveliest thing you can to her. And don't hold back. Be gushing and enthusiastic with this self-love and kindness. The more fabulous, the better.

Write your compliment down each day, and at the end of the week go back and read them all out loud. The energy of a week's worth of compliments can have a profound impact on your mood and self-esteem, and you can revisit

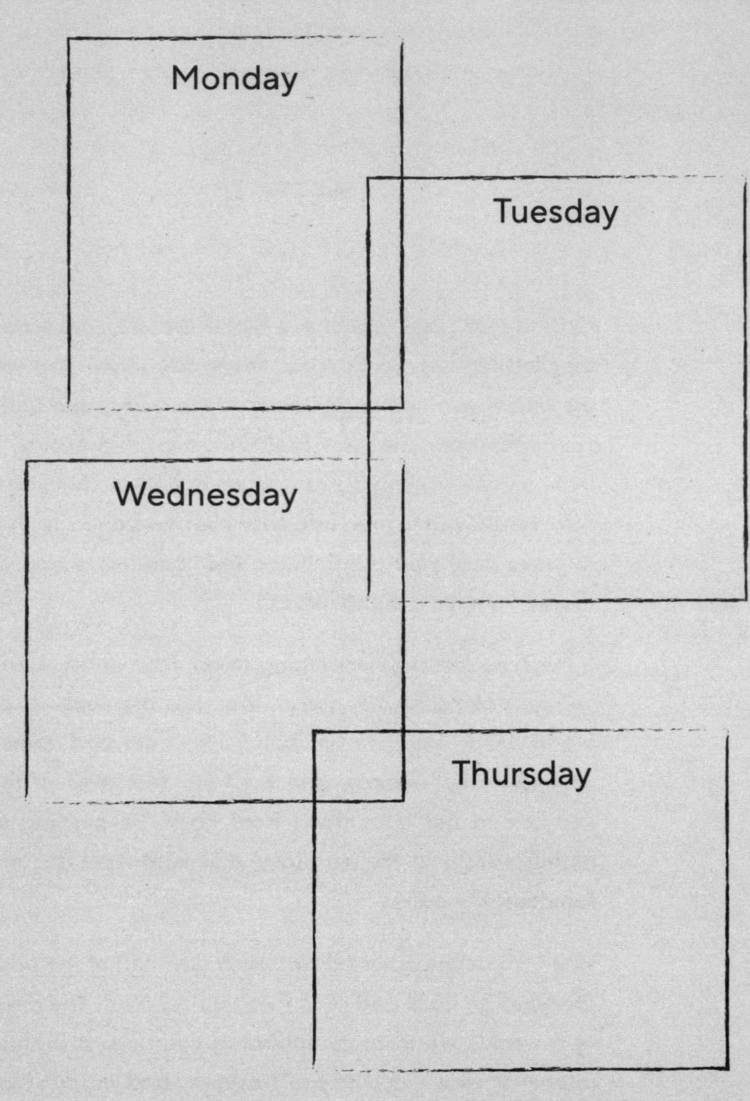
Monday
Tuesday
Wednesday
Thursday

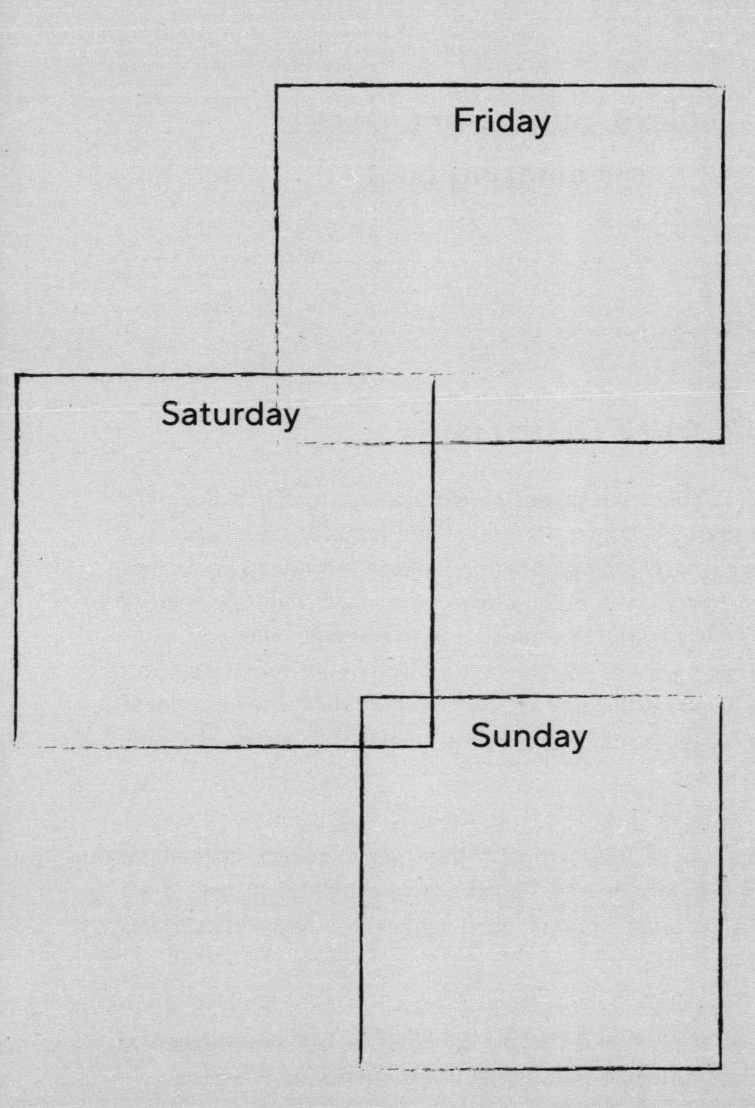
Friday
Saturday
Sunday

I love, nurture and enjoy my amazing body

IGNITING YOUR INTUITION

We often hear about the power of intuition or 'mother's gut'. We touched on this in The First 48 Hours (see page 36) but actually, I think there's so much *coping* going on in those first twelve weeks that it can take a little time to acclimatise and connect with this internal GPS, which is why I want to explore it in more depth with you here. Now first of all, I want to say that even if you're not somebody who identifies as being particularly intuitive, you will definitely have come into contact with your intuition over the course of your life, probably many times in fact.

Our intuition is a bit like a muscle that needs looking after. If we neglect it, it deteriorates and becomes more difficult to use. If we exercise it, it becomes stronger and makes our life and activities easier to enjoy.

Developing your intuition is completely possible, and can make one of the most tangible differences to your experience as a mother.

So what actually *is* intuition? People will describe their experiences of intuition differently, but essentially I want you to think of it as an inner sense and the ability to understand or decide on something without conscious reasoning. It is a feeling that you may be able to identify in your stomach, your mind or your heart – a sense that you know what is right for you in a particular moment, without something obvious or explicit confirming it. With motherhood especially, where there are a lot of external voices telling us what we *should* be doing or what things are *meant* to look/feel like, it can be incredibly insightful and empowering when we learn to turn down that outside noise and focus our attention inwards.

The idea of igniting your intuition is all about awakening to your most authentic self and the life that feels most aligned with your heart and soul. Motherhood is one of the most personal and profound journeys you will ever be on, and I believe you have a choice – to exist alongside it or to fully embrace its magic and make it your own.

In the early days with my first child, I know I did a lot of existing/hanging on/internet-scouring/copying/comparing myself to others because I was so far removed from my own ideas and intuition. It wasn't until certain events and experiences unfolded, and I had a sense, in hindsight, of 'why did I do/not do that?', that I realised I was missing a trick by not paying attention to this invisible compass inside me. As time went on, I risked listening to it and was constantly taken aback by how much easier and more enjoyable it was making motherhood, and my life in general. Listening to this intuition goes beyond knowing what's right for your baby. It applies to all aspects of our lives, and recognising the contribution of your intuition to life's bigger picture is really important. When we tune in to what feels right for us in *our* situation or set-up, we can make more informed decisions that are better suited to improving our own personal sense of well-being and happiness. This isn't going to happen overnight, but I have worked to actively exercise this muscle, and I'm excited to teach you how to do the same.

ACTIVITY

SPONTANEOUS CREATIONS

This is a seemingly simple exercise that offers a super-effective way to start igniting your intuition. This inner wisdom appears most strongly when we make space for it, and that means being relaxed and calm – something that I think we can all agree isn't always easy when you're looking after small people! This activity is going to introduce you to the art of relaxed thoughts, and wonderfully, requires no conscious effort whatsoever. All I want you to do is set a timer on your phone for one minute and practise the Calm Breath (see page 33) for that time. When you have done that, I want you to pick up a pen or pencil, set the timer for five minutes, and write whatever comes into your head in the space overleaf, until the timer goes off. It doesn't have to be about you, motherhood, this activity, or anything currently in your consciousness. Literally let the pen take you, and follow the natural

path of your mind without questioning where you're going.

Don't read back what you've written straight away. That's when we can start to overthink, become critical or consciously analyse our thoughts, and this often leads us away from our gut feelings. Instead, come back to what you've written in two or three days, and see if you can connect to anything you wrote about in that five-minute space. Did you identify a certain feeling in what you wrote – fear, pride, excitement? Did you wander somewhere quite abstract that can be unpicked as the things going on in your head? Did you learn something about yourself? At first, you may not, but if you practise doing this regularly you may well start to notice a greater sense of ease around your thoughts and feelings, and a closer alignment to what you are writing, how you are feeling, and what is happening in your life.

If you don't enjoy writing or can't connect with the spontaneous flow of it, you could try drawing instead. Everyone has creative leanings (just the way you choose to express yourself reveals your natural creativity, even if you wouldn't identify as someone overtly creative), and you want this exercise to involve the most comfortable form of expression for you. Remember that just like with motherhood, there is no right or wrong here. This is about finding *your* way and celebrating the uniqueness of *you*.

To begin with, try to do this two or three times a week. If you think about it, it's only six minutes of activity because it requires (actually, it relies upon) no forward planning! It's also a really good one to do if ever your thoughts are feeling jumbled, if you're being bombarded with differing opinions, or if you're having trouble identifying how you really feel about a particular issue.

While this exercise is a very practical and direct way of exercising your intuition muscle, there are many, many other things you can do to help support your maternal awakening and to incorporate these learnings into a celebrated part of your identity. I think we have a tendency to overcomplicate things like meditation or mindfulness, when in fact at the heart of this growth is quiet, space and the skill and patience to listen. This will take time, but remember it is an ongoing journey. You are learning and growing every day as a mother, and there is no race or finish line. Finding your intuition isn't always going to feel like a straightforward path either. There will be twists and turns while you work out how to tune in your emotional aerial, and that's to be embraced as part of the fun! Here are some more ideas for how you can gently incorporate this practice into life with your baby, and exercise your intuition daily.

THREE SIMPLE QUESTIONS

Asking yourself these three simple questions can work to quickly put you in touch with your subconscious experience in any given moment. Personally, I like to ask myself these three questions when I wake up in the morning – normally after I'm out of bed and have had a cup of tea. I'll often do it when I'm brushing my teeth or having a shower, as these things give me a few quiet moments to ponder them without distraction. The questions are:

How am I feeling?

What is this feeling telling me?

What do I need today?

Give it a go when you're feeling foggy or anxious – it can really become a sure-fire way to benefit from even the trickiest of emotions. Why? Because every single thing you feel and experience is telling you something. It's your job to listen, and this is a great place to start.

INTUITIVE ADVENTURE

How many times do we hear 'do this with intention' or 'do that with purpose' – but what if I tell you that the opposite can be beneficial, too? We are often so busy and have so much to do (especially as mums) that we run around ticking off our to-do list without much sense of our experience of how we've actually done it. How many times have you driven somewhere and not remembered the route you took, or forgotten what day/year it is? Again, if you're feeling lost, overwhelmed, or completely distracted by what everyone else is doing, take yourself on an intuitive adventure.

Pop your baby in their buggy or in the car seat and go out for either a walk or a drive. The only two rules are that you're not allowed to think about where you're going, and you're not allowed to incorporate any jobs along the way – no picking up milk, no popping to the post office – you are out purely to follow the calling of your present thoughts. Notice where they take you, ignite your senses and tune in to what is around you. What can you see? What can you hear? What does the ground feel like beneath your feet? The closer and more quietly we lean into our surroundings, the more likely we are to hear the call of our authentic experience and intuition.

DAYDREAM BELIEVER

Hands up if you had some really weird dreams when you were pregnant. Thought so. This is generally thought to be down to our fluctuating hormones when we're expecting, but remember that it can take a while for your hormones to resettle after your baby is born, too. With that in mind, you may notice that you continue to have more vivid dreams in your first year of motherhood, and they can actually prove to be incredibly insightful and helpful in moving you closer to your maternal wisdom and instincts. Keep a notepad and pen next to your bed, and when you wake up in the night (for feeds, resettling your baby or needing the toilet), jot down anything you can remember about your dreams. You can do this in the morning too, but it's a nice way to make use of that broken sleep! The next day, read back over what you've written and try to align your thoughts with what the dream is telling you. This is rarely going to be a literal translation, so try to think broadly and about what message the dream is giving you and what feelings it prompts in you.

CREATIVE OUTLET

When was the last time you did something creative? So many of our leisure interests or hobbies fall by the wayside when we become mothers, but it doesn't need to be that way. When we use the creative parts of our brain, we can achieve a more relaxed and meditative state, and this can in turn move us closer to our intuition and gut feelings. Get yourself a small, blank notepad and dedicate five minutes a week to creative output. This could be anything – doodling, sketching, painting, writing, colouring – whatever most appeals to you, and again, just create without purpose, for creation's sake. Afterwards, observe your creations and notice how you feel. Did your mind wander anywhere unexpected? Does your body or breathing feel any different? Recognising the benefits of these activities means you're more likely to do them again.

While we definitely want to be mindful of always looking to other people for the answers, we can learn how to use outside sources to support, inform and grow our intuition. When you turn to the internet, books, or other people for help and information, try to see it as getting lots of ideas that will inform your own decision-making rather than doing it for you. There is so rarely a one-size-fits-all way of doing anything motherhood-related, so keep an open mind and give yourself time to digest new information and ideas.

Similarly, I know that resisting comparisons with other people is so much easier said than done. Again though, try to use your community as a source of inspiration and thought expansion, rather than as a conveyor-belt method you need to blanket-apply to your own life. We all have a unique frame of reference and set of personal circumstances, so practise observing information and ideas without having to instantly apply them. When we give these sources of inspiration space and consideration, we become better at taking what we need and leaving what we don't, and this is all part of finding your *own* way at your *own* pace.

EMBRACING YOUR NEW SENSE OF SELF

Having felt like you've been leaping over the hurdles of sleep deprivation on the heels of your hormones during your baby's first few months on Earth, it's likely that around this time, you will slowly start to feel like things are settling – on a hormonal level at least. Your baby may be sleeping for slightly longer (or at least more predictable) periods, you are likely to begin feeling more confident in how you're feeding your baby, and you will be more in tune with what their little noises and cues mean.

> There is a sense of coming home to yourself, and while that might look a bit different to what you knew before, these new layers of yourself are something to embrace, celebrate and lean into.

You are doing such a brilliant job of responding to your baby, and I want to help you to honour and enjoy all of these wonderful new things you are learning about yourself too.

When we emerge from our fourth trimester, get to know and understand our baby a little more, and begin to settle into our own ideas about motherhood, questions around our own identity can start surfacing and we often ask ourselves 'who am I becoming?'. For the last three months or so, most of your time, thoughts and energy will have centred around meeting your baby's physical demands and emotional needs, and while that will obviously continue, there will slowly start to be more space for giving back to yourself.

Before we become mothers, our identity is often focused around our profession, our relationships or social life and our extra interests and skills, and while these things might have been on pause, it's okay to acknowledge that they are still important to you. Similarly, you might be so fully immersed in life with your baby that they don't seem to matter, and that's okay too; but either way you will hopefully be homing in on what's important to you based on where you're at in this moment.

Many of us have a lot of preconceived ideas of what parenthood is going to look like – what our baby might be like, what kind of mother we will be, and what life will look like when our family expands. It's not unusual for things to unfold in a completely different way to what we've imagined, and I want to invite you to embrace this new reality without placing too much pressure on what you thought things might look like.

ACTIVITY

MOTHERHOOD MOOD BOARD

You may well be familiar with the concept of a mood board – maybe you've created one professionally or as part of a personal development journey. Maybe you wrote a birth plan while you were pregnant, and then learned first-hand that our best-laid plans can sometimes go astray – which is why I always suggest that birth *preferences* are a better way of approaching things. Similarly, a motherhood mood board allows for our thoughts and feelings around motherhood to grow, adapt and evolve as our experience does.

In this activity, I want you to consider and seek out inspiration that aligns with your desired experience of motherhood. You may already have ideas around what kind of mother you want to be, and this will help you to hone in on those things and explore them more.

Maybe you want to be structured, child-led, play-based, parent-led, maybe you want to encourage lots of books, maybe you want to do lots of explorative play, maybe you want to be in control of what your child eats or maybe you want to let them control this at their own pace. There are so many things here that we may never have even considered before we had our children, but acknowledging the ideas that you connect with can really help you nurture and lean into that part of yourself.

Use magazines, books, poems, photos, song lyrics or quotes for inspiration, and gradually collate clippings of these ideas. On a sheet of paper, start arranging these visual ideas and then stick them down so that the sheet appeals to you aesthetically. If you use a big sheet, you can keep adding to it and the more you find, the more you will be inspired to explore and embrace your maternal identity. When we are surrounded by so much noise about what motherhood *should* look like, I always find that this activity offers such a welcome breather to nurture our own ideas and desires instead of being influenced by external opinions and pressure.

When you've made your mood board, keep it somewhere you can see it (and even add to it) often, as a way of centring yourself in your own ideas at a moment's notice.

Let's remember too, that while it can be great to explore this new part of your self, this can also be a time when you might want to invite back parts of yourself that you are missing or craving. You haven't got to choose between your old self and your new self, but rather celebrate the combination of both, and find a new kind of normal – a celebration of every step of your journey so far.

Once you've been catapulted into the intensity of motherhood and its all-encompassing demands, it can feel like you're a long way from what you used to love, but you're really never that far away – she/you/her remain right there inside. If you feel ready to start reconnecting with these parts of yourself, why not try asking yourself the following questions:

What do I love?

If I had two hours to myself, what would I do?

What from my pre-baby life made me feel confident and good about myself?

By exploring the answers to these questions (in your mind or on paper), you can start incorporating what *made* you tick into what *makes* you tick, and that's what embracing this new chapter is all about. Not all or nothing, but a sprinkling of many things.

Here's an example: Let's say you were previously a member of a choir, or you used to attend a dance/exercise class. Sure, committing to a regular group activity right now is probably not feeling so feasible, but how can you bring it into your motherhood journey in an easy and enjoyable way? Often the block in accessing these parts of ourselves is in our mind. We make excuses for why we can't do something any more, but actually, it's just about being creative and adaptable. Think about it. You could play a song you love while having a shower – sing it at the top of your lungs and notice how good it feels to connect with your voice again – or, while baby sleeps or is being taken care of by someone else, put a dance or exercise video on YouTube, have a stretch and express yourself! Things might not look exactly the same, but you can certainly begin to bring familiar joy and expressions of yourself back into your onward journey, and I promise you'll feel amazing (and relieved!) for it.

When we do something we love, have fun, laugh or connect, we're producing those all-important endorphins that lift our mood and make us feel positive and calm. And that goes for our babies too. When we feel more happy and at ease, we inevitably share that energy with our little ones too, and they feed off the way we feel.

FINDING YOUR TRIBE

While we have touched on the topic of who you're going to be leaning on during those early days of life with your little one – new-mum friends included – I think it's a good idea to take a deeper delve into the relationships you're likely to find and firm up over the coming months and years. It's likely that by the time you become a mother, you'll already have a trusted group of friends from your journey through life to this point. Whether these are friends from school, university, travelling, work or hobbies, friendships are normally a big part of our lives from early on. Whether you have a partner or are a solo parent, our friends are a source of support, comfort and joy – our companions in the good times and our confidantes in the trickier ones. It is natural that in life we sometimes lose old friends and often make new ones, but we hope to keep a sacred few close to us until we're old. It's also normal for some of our relationships to ebb and flow, but the truest of friendships will survive the crashes of life's bigger waves and always return to the shore.

We have seen so far in this book that when we take the plunge into starting a family, so much changes. Whether we have a partner to share the ups and downs with, are well supported by family, or are embarking on this adventure on our own, our lifestyle and priorities can shift in a heartbeat, and this can inevitably take its toll on all of our relationships, including those with our friends. While that doesn't mean you have to ditch your current friends, it can mean you temporarily take a step away from your usual social circles, and that can leave you feeling isolated and lonely. As such, I'm inviting you to consider your journey into motherhood as a wonderful opportunity to extend your support network by adding to it women who are having similar experiences.

That said, making new friends can feel like a huge effort, and one that when you're sleep-deprived you may well think isn't worth the energy. Let's focus on the positive though and come at this from an empowering and everyday perspective. After all, this doesn't have to be about joint birthday parties and group family holidays for years to come, but rather, the day-to-day support that finding your tribe of supportive, like-minded women with little ones of a similar age will offer up in spades.

Why do I need new friends?

Maybe you're one of the lucky few who has happened to time having babies to coincide with your besties, but in case you haven't, here are some reasons why finding your tribe in this new realm can be brilliantly advantageous for everyone involved:

- **Having people who can relate to the emotional tides of motherhood**

  There's no denying that one of the biggest challenges of modern motherhood is the shift it presents by way of our identity, confidence and purpose. It's very easy to lose ourselves in the all-consuming nature of early motherhood, and it can be frightening to feel like we're slipping away from the structures we have always known. While everyone around us seems to be skipping along in life as normal, we are spending more time at home, with much less adult company than we're probably used to, and constantly trying to adapt to and meet the changing needs of our baby. While the joy, pride and love can feel completely unparalleled, it's fair to say that there will also be times where we're left doubting ourselves or feeling lonely. Having someone who can identify with these feelings and who can truly empathise with the emotional transition you're going through can be so helpful in not losing your marbles and knowing that you're not alone in these ups and downs.

- **Enjoying adult company on maternity leave**

  If I had a pound for every time I've heard someone refer to maternity leave as 'time off', I'd be a rich woman. Maternity leave is just a different kind of work – one that works on the currency of love without the traditional benefits of a lunch break or sick pay. Maternity leave is full-on and relentless. It's also precious and sacred and wonderful, and it can be even more of that stuff when we are able to enjoy and navigate it with supportive people. Days at home snuggled up with your baby can be gorgeous and love-fuelled, but some days can be draining, disorientating and, dare I say it, boring at times too! If you're used to working with other people, you may find yourself really missing adult interaction and conversation, and finding like-minded mums to meet up with can be a real lifeline on that front. Sure, you might kick off conversation with an update on night-wakings or a question about poo, but I bet you'll soon find yourselves talking about things that are way more interesting as well, and realise that you haven't lost that sense of self after all!

- **Bounce boards for babies of a similar age**

  No matter how many baby books you read, there's nothing quite like getting to know other mums and babies for that reassurance that every single baby grows and develops in their own unique way. My second son – according to Dr Google – was slow to sit up and crawl, but actually having seen that he was one of five babies just doing things at different times within my group of mum friends meant I didn't worry, and quickly realised that they were all learning tiny different skills in varying orders, just like we do as adults! Babies aren't robots, and when you get the chance to observe and talk about the nuances of their development with similarly interested mums, it can offer such comfort in those early months of change.

- **Practical support when you need it most**

  There's no denying that when you have a baby, you could also do with about six extra pairs of hands at times. Mothers have this special skill for multi-tasking/balancing/carrying that is basically a superpower, but even so, there are days when a helping hand is most welcome. One of the greatest joys for me of finding mum friends is the practical support we can offer each other and how much it is valued and appreciated. There have been times when a friend has picked up my older son from school, or brought round food when I was suffering from mastitis, and it has honestly been incredible. This can be a blessing on a more day-to-day level too. Perhaps you and a friend could take turns having each other's baby for an hour so that you can go for a haircut or get a bit of exercise – something that makes you feel like you again. There's something really special about knowing these people get it and have your back, and that you'd so readily return the favour for them too, meaning nothing's ever done out of obligation or with any expectation or emotional cost.

Now, when you're on the outside looking in, it can be easy to see groups of mums pushing buggies or having coffee and think that everyone has made friends except for you. That is not the case. I repeat, that is not the case. Every mum I've ever met has felt nervous about connecting with other mums and putting themselves out there. While lots will take the leap before baby arrives by joining an antenatal class and bagging some mates along the way, remember that plenty of women don't do this, and you are not the odd one out if that's you. Add to this the fact that not everyone has a baby at the same time as their friends, or has a network nearby, and you'll be amazed at how many new mums are feeling exactly the same way as you.

How do I make new friends?

Whether you are a social butterfly or struggle with the confidence to forge new friendships, believe me when I say that you can do this. Most mums I know are longing to meet other smart, supportive women, so you are all in this together, and taking the leap to put yourself out there may just be one of the most rewarding steps you take on this journey. Here are some gentle ideas for meeting new mum friends – give them a go when you're feeling ready!

Go along to your local playgroup

While some baby classes may be expensive or require a minimum time commitment, there are often free or purse-friendly playgroups run in church halls or community centres. If you have a local Facebook page, keep your eyes peeled for what's on near you, or ask your health visitor or local children's centre if they can direct you towards any groups. There will usually be toys laid out for different-aged babies and toddlers, and you'll be able to grab a cup of tea and a biscuit and stay for however long you want to. It will be full of people in the same boat as you, and can be a really relaxed way to get chatting to new people.

Join a postnatal well-being class

If you're at the stage where you want to start filling up your cup again and making time to nurture and nourish yourself, you may well be considering finding a postnatal fitness or well-being class. There are all sorts of set-ups nowadays – from Buggy Fit to baby-wearing exercise classes, postnatal Pilates and mum/baby yoga. Going along to something like this will not only give you the opportunity to build your physical strength and confidence, but may well also introduce you to other mums who feel the same way.

A pinch of salt and social media

While I always think that social media should be approached with caution as a new mum (remember that you're seeing people's highlight reels and not always real life!), it can offer a genuine lifeline to women who don't have a physical network around them. Follow other mothers who you find encouraging and empowering, and maybe you'll be inspired by ways they've found to meet people. It may even introduce you to other local mums who are online too.

Swings and roundabouts (and coffee)

Playgrounds and parks are a brilliant way to meet other parents, especially as your baby gets a little older and can enjoy things like swings and slides. I have met so many other mums while walking around the park during nap time (or queuing for coffee!), and it offers a relaxed opportunity to strike up a conversation while enjoying some fresh air and open space, especially if you can see that their baby is of a similar age. If you hit it off then why not suggest grabbing a coffee and going for a walk, or meeting in the park again another time? There's no pressure, and I bet you'll get a real boost from sparking up a conversation and enjoying how good that feels.

*

One thing I want to add here is to bring in that intuition that we talked about back on page 168. When your intuition is switched on, you will begin to notice who your energy increases and decreases around, or in other words who makes you feel great and who leaves you feeling depleted. If someone is making you feel bad or unsure of yourself, or like you have to be someone you're not, then don't be afraid to remove yourself and protect your own headspace. Your friends should make you feel good about yourself, and make you feel like *you*. The ones who don't are not your people.

ACTIVITY

THE GOOD FRIEND GUIDE

Something to bear in mind if you're looking for friends at an antenatal class is that to a point you're simply there with this group of women because you all happen to be having babies at the same time. Sometimes that's as far as the common ground goes, which isn't always going to make for the most robust or rewarding friendships.

In this activity I want you to identify what being a good friend means to you, both in terms of what you offer as a friend and what you'd like to receive from a friend. On the page opposite, you'll see an illustration of two women. One is you, and the other is your dream mum mate.

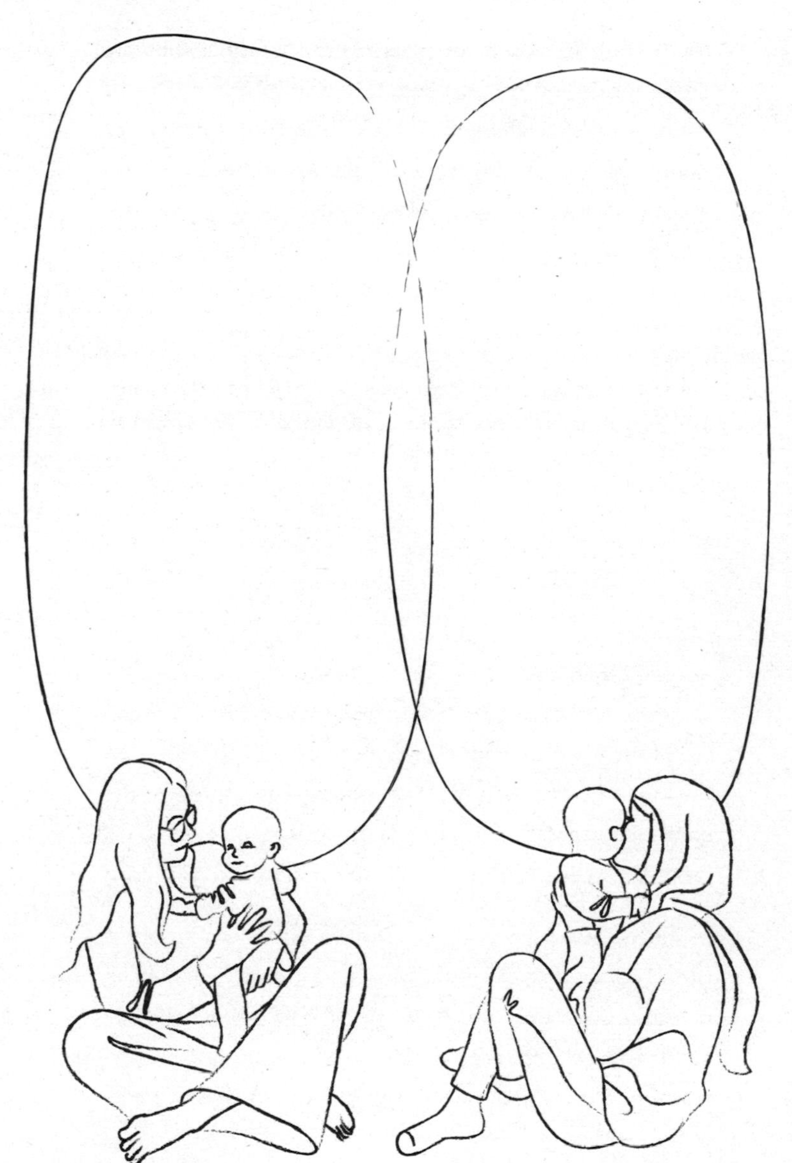

In the bubble above you, identify the qualities that you think make you a good friend and label them. Do the same for the qualities you'd look for in your dream mum mate. So it might be a good listener, someone who is funny, someone who likes music/baking/exercise/reading.

Identifying the qualities that represent a fulfilling friendship will help you to find it in others, and acknowledging what you bring to your social relationships will boost your confidence on that front too!

A FINAL THOUGHT

This can be a really exciting and rewarding time in your motherhood journey and it can be easy to emerge, after the fourth trimester, and want to throw yourself full-pelt into the next stages of your baby's development; but remember, it's still okay to go slow.

There's no rush to reach milestones or achieve anything in particular; and you and your baby are still getting used to each other, and learning a lot. You are learning each other's languages, becoming more familiar with each other's nuances and building trusting connectedness every day.

Don't be disheartened if you're finding things tough. It **is** tough, and in the grand scheme of motherhood, this is still very early days in your adventure. Even though it doesn't always feel like it, you are learning and growing as a mother all the time, and blossoming brilliantly into the mother your little one needs you to be.

Try to keep checking in with yourself each day – notice how you're feeling and recognise when you need to top up your cup and take better care of yourself. These strong loving bonds that we want to share with our children start with us, so remember that by looking after yourself, you are also caring for those around you. Have a go at the exercises in this section whenever you need to be reminded of just how capable and brilliant you are, and don't be afraid to lean into your vulnerabilities and celebrate your strengths.

Above all, keep going and remember that you are enough, just the way you are.

I accept, embrace and celebrate every part of who I am

SPACE TO REFLECT

SPACE TO REFLECT

PART FOUR

ONWARDS AND UPWARDS:

EMBRACING THE FUTURE (6 MONTHS+)

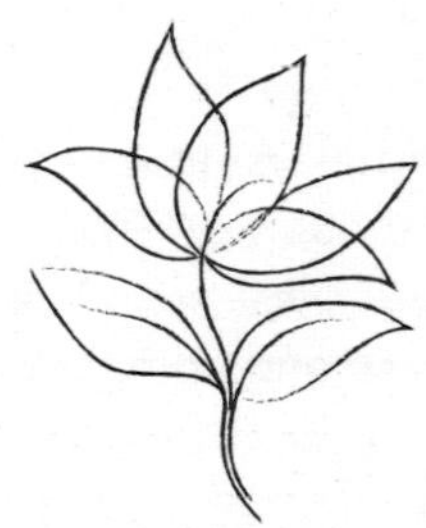

After spending half a year getting to know your baby, you will hopefully be feeling more confident and comfortable with how life is evolving. Even if that's not the case yet, maybe you can notice the small steps that are moving you in the direction of this feeling. It could be something as simple as feeling less triggered or panicked in stressful situations, that you're sleeping better, or that you are managing to cope and react more calmly when challenges come your way. Be careful not to miss these subtle indicators of your growth. It may still feel like life's all over the place at times, but I bet if you look more closely, you'll realise how far you've come since the day you met your baby. The shocks-to-the-system and rollercoaster of emotions are hopefully starting to settle as you adapt to your new kind of normal – one that you are becoming adept at navigating, even when it's hard. I know I keep saying it, but quite frankly, why not? You should be SO proud of yourself.

It's likely that at the half-year mark, your baby may be starting to show some signs of falling into a more natural routine in terms of sleep and awake time. They are likely to be having two naps a day (morning and after lunch), and this brings with it a very welcome return of some predictability and structure to our days. I remember feeling with both my babies that things began to feel a bit calmer and easier once we hit this six-month mark – almost as if I'd completed my motherhood probation period and was now trusted to get on with the job!

While this can be a welcome relief for lots of us, we should know by now that every up also has its down – such is the ever-changing equilibrium of the maternal journey. This newfound confidence can lead us to overlook the care we still need to be directing back towards ourselves, and the kindness and compassion we must continue to show ourselves when things go off-piste. I really want to encourage you to keep seeing this as a journey, and one where you are learning and growing as a mother every day. While things are likely to feel more familiar and you more competent, we all still have our down days and it's important to keep that cup topped up and our emotional well-being in check.

In this section, we're going to explore the ongoing journey with yourself, your network and your baby, and I'm going to be giving you lots of activities that will help to keep you calm and connected along the way. I've said it before and I'll say it again – there is no right or wrong way to do this, and leaning into the elements of discovery you'll continue to stumble upon is one of the greatest gifts the coming months and years have to offer.

YOUR SELF

IDENTITY HOMECOMING

By now, you can probably relate to the sense of those first six months of your baby's life as being a physical and emotional whirlwind. You and your baby have been learning so much, finding your own way, exploring the world around you and adjusting into a rhythm that works for you and your family. It is such a consuming period of motherhood – for obvious reasons – and we've already touched on that idea of having to park a big part of ourselves while we relentlessly meet our baby's every need. Don't underestimate what a big deal that is. I know we have little choice over it, but the commitment, guts and love it takes to nurture someone so unconditionally is the most incredible thing I've ever come across. You get so little breathing room, thinking space or me-time that it's little wonder that, when it starts to reappear, it can seem bewildering, unfamiliar, and at times overwhelming.

I strongly remember this sense of not knowing what to do with myself when I started to get pockets of time back because my baby was asleep or being taken care of by someone else. I'll never forget my eldest's first morning at childcare. It was only a two-hour session and I sat in the car and stared out of the window for the whole time – I was literally paralysed by the offering of time to myself. Whether or not childcare is on your immediate horizon, maybe you can relate to that feeling of not knowing how to give back to yourself when your baby starts having a regular nap, or not knowing where to start with reconnecting to your identity, and that's exactly what I want to address here.

Feeling a disconnect between what you consider to be your old and your new identities is widespread among mothers, and it's definitely something I've had many conversations about with friends and clients over the years. So if you're feeling a bit lost or overwhelmed by the idea of finding yourself again, you are most certainly not alone. Feelings of uncertainty around your identity could manifest as not being sure of your place or purpose in the world, not knowing what your future might look like, feeling discontent or distanced from things you used to love, or even feeling a sense of grief for your old life. All of those experiences are valid and normal. Having a baby is not an everyday occurrence. It's a life-changing, world-spinning ride, and it's understandable that it takes us a while to get our feet back on the ground again.

If you've been getting stuck into some of the activities in this book so far, you will hopefully be starting to feel a sense of reflection and reconnection with who you are and what you want your experience of motherhood to be like. If you had a go at the Motherhood Mood Board exercise (see page 179), now might be a good time to revisit your creation. Hopefully you are beginning to feel calmer, more confident, and better equipped to approach your days with clarity and compassion towards yourself and your home unit. Now can also be a brilliant time to really invite more parts of your parked self *back*, and embrace with open arms how this fits into all the new bits of you, too. What you're taking forward now is a deeper sense of self: the layers that have always been there and the new parts that unfold and evolve as your journey goes on. Invite them all in. Notice what makes you feel good, and lean into it with all you have. Why not revisit your Breather Branches too (see page 42), and visualise the motherhood journey like the inner trunk of a tree, where each layer of growth represents your expanding strength and wisdom.

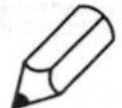

ACTIVITY

ALL THE THINGS I LOVE

We have explored an early-days version of this activity already, but now that your baby is getting a little older you may feel you can be a bit more ambitious in the ways you rediscover your interests and passions. In this activity I want to give you an opportunity to reflect on all the things you loved about your life before you became a mum. I don't normally suggest compartmentalising our pre-/post-baby selves because I think it's an ever-changing growth process that should be celebrated as a whole, but in this instance it can be helpful to get back in touch with the parts of ourselves that might feel missed or perhaps just far away.

First of all, I want you to write down a few things in your life that you enjoy reminiscing about. Think about three things you've done that made you feel really alive and engaged. This could be anything from travelling, to being part of a team or involved in a personal or professional project, to going out with friends and properly letting your hair down. If you're struggling to even identify these moments, try revisiting those ideas in your Motherhood Mood Board on page 179. Keep in mind that it doesn't have to be anything too specific. It could relate to a broader life experience, like being in your workplace or on holiday.

On the page overleaf, write down what that experience was and, using the Calm Breath technique (see page 33), regulate your breathing, close your eyes if that feels comfortable, and take yourself back to that time in your mind's eye. Try to remember what things looked like, how you felt and who you were with. Engage your senses in the experience and just let yourself rest and observe that place for a few minutes.

When you've done that, use the space to answer and explore these questions. Your answers might not come straight away, but you can just jot down words or feelings if that's easier.

What did you enjoy about this activity or experience?

For example: if it's a sport, was it being part of a team, improving your technique, being physically active etc.

How did you feel after this activity or experience?

For example: relaxed, energised, tired, proud, relieved, insightful.

Why did you stop this activity or experience?

For example: outgrowing a group, getting bored, not having time to commit to hobbies, changing location, peer pressure etc.

What was the single best thing about this experience, or what do you miss most about it?

For example: the learning experience, the sense of camaraderie, being able to master a technique etc.

When you've answered these questions, take your time reflecting on what you've written. Often we are quick to write off things we used to love because we assume we won't have time for them any more, but actually, if we focus on the specifics of what appealed and engaged us, we can get a clearer sense of what that reveals about our identity and find ways to bring those pleasures into our current life picture.

Let me give you an example. Let's say you really enjoyed dancing when you were younger. By answering the questions above, you've identified that you enjoyed having a way to express yourself and an outlet for stress, that you felt a sense of pleasure and confidence afterwards, that you stopped because you had less free time and money, or because your friendships changed, and that you miss having that opportunity for letting your hair down and enjoying yourself. Now you can look at those personal feelings and figure out how you can bring a dose of them back to life.

You may not be able to tick all the boxes straight away, but you can definitely start to consider or even forward-plan ideas that might put you back in touch with this sense of identity and personal enjoyment. If it's dancing you missed, could you find a dance class you can take your baby along to (or there are even toddler raves, believe it or not!), or even just put on some music when your little one's gone to bed and have a dance around the kitchen? Or if what you loved about dancing was the sense of mastering a technique, but you can't regularly commit to lessons or leaving the house, could you look at an online or home-study course in something like calligraphy? It's something you could do at home, maybe for half an hour a couple of times a week, and practise at your own pace. You would get a creative outlet, a single focus, and the opportunity to master a new technique; and you'll be surprised at how effectively something seemingly unrelated can put you back in touch with your identity and lead it lovingly forward. Try to keep an open mind even if the things you miss feel unattainable at the moment. For instance, if you loved travelling pre-kids – why not think about exploring a local city and being a tourist in your own town for the day, or even taking your baby along to an art gallery or exhibition? It could be a brilliant way to reignite that interest and have a lovely day with your little one at the same time.

Give it a go. If you are returning to work around now, this activity can be a brilliant way to use your commute, or a quiet moment in your lunch break. It might not work for every activity you reflect on, but if you start with three, I know you'll quickly identify small snippets of your personality that may initially seem far away, and that is one great big step in the right direction.

BALANCING PRODUCTIVITY AND REST

A lot of the pressure we put on ourselves, whether we're first-time or more seasoned mothers, comes from the expectation we feel from the world around us – a world we're now beginning to re-engage with. With the prevalence of social media, we are constantly consuming a showreel of people's achievements – mums crafting, tidying, exercising, cooking and starting a business on the side – when we can barely find the time to eat a sandwich. It can lead to us feeling like we should always be doing more, that we are never enough, and that we are inadequate or lazy. I find this idea so upsetting, because while it's just not true, it can also be really damaging to our perspective of productivity and worth, and the ability to grant ourselves permission to rest.

The reality is that motherhood is a full-time job (perhaps one you're now doing alongside another full-time job) and whether you have returned to work, will be soon, or are continuing to look after your baby full-time, you are doing completely enough. We don't have to add more on top of that – it's fine of course if we *want or need* to, but it's important to reflect on whether that impulse comes from what you genuinely want and feel, or the broader societal narrative.

I'd like you to consider for a moment that everything you are doing is outstanding. You are achieving more than you ever have (even though it might not be so obvious or tangible) and you are making one of the most important, profound and valuable contributions to society (if you're feeling any doubt about this, revisit A Mama's Worth... on page 149). As the months and years go by and you wonder what you've been doing, look into your child's eyes and notice how they smile or how those eyes soften or meet your gaze. You are a constant source of love and security right now, and it's so important that you take this belief into your onward journey for two reasons. The first is so that you stop doubting yourself – that you feel in your heart the worth of your work and know that whatever phase you're in isn't permanent. The second is so that you grant yourself permission to rest without needing to offset it against tangible achievements. Let me explain.

If we accomplish a recognised activity or achievement – let's say earning a degree or running a marathon – it's obvious to everyone that loads of work and preparation has gone into it and that we are deserving of a rest or downtime. If we are marathon training, we have rest days between run days; or we'll take breaks from studying to switch off and relax. This is a given – something that keeps us going and that can be readily recognised as essential to our achievements and our well-being. Contrast this against the perception of life as a mother – that whole idea of 'just a mum' for instance that we talked about back on page 147. We're *just* at home all day or we *just* work part-time. We're *just* holding baby. We're *just* playing. We're *just* tidying up. We're *just just just*. I know you will have heard those things at one point or another, and it's essential that we can recognise that they're merely narratives locked in our subconscious.

This mentality can be even more prevalent among women who return to the workplace. We can feel as if we're in some kind of productivity limbo – rushing around and feeling like not enough of us is anywhere – so it's really important to show yourself some compassion as life continues to evolve and change.

So how do we move past this? What can we do? Well, it's much like our preparation for birth. We need to perform an audit on our subconscious mind so that we can work out what beliefs are really ours and which ones aren't. Then we can reprogramme our subconscious with a loving acknowledgement of our hard work, which in turn will make it easier for us to embrace our entitlement to rest, *without* feeling guilty.

Achieving a balance between productivity and rest is not easy, but with the right mental approach it can definitely be done and I promise you, it is life-changing. As soon as you can start acknowledging rest as essential to your output, everything shifts and those destructive sprinklings of guilt and resentment start to disappear. It's not going to happen overnight, but incorporating this next activity into your daily or weekly routine will be a huge step in the right direction.

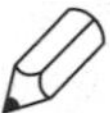

ACTIVITY

TA-DAH LIST

We are all familiar with to-do lists. They might be in our head, in notebooks, on our phone or scribbled onto scraps of paper at the bottom of our bag, but at one time or another, we'll have made plenty. The idea of having tangible jobs and being able to tick them off can be mentally satisfying, and while that's no bad thing, it pretty much flies out of the window when we have babies to look after. Suddenly there's no set schedule, no rhyme or reason to each day, and our plans become predominantly dictated by someone who can't speak.

Rather than start your day with a to-do list, I want you to now end your day with a ta-dah list. Writing down all of the things we've done in a day – no matter how small or insignificant they seem – can give you such incredible perspective on how much you really are achieving, even if (or especially when) it goes unseen. If you've gone back to work full- or part-time, this can prove to be an even more valuable exercise; your work days may well feel productive and ordered, so try this activity both when you've been at work and when you've spent the day with your baby. Your two lists might look pretty different, but it's a great opportunity to identify your output in different capacities, even when some are more tangible than others.

On the following page, pop the date at the top and then use the bullet points to write down every single thing you do in one day. You might find these hard to recall or remember by the end of the day, so to start with I want you to write them down as you go along. It's really important that you include everything here. Don't think 'that doesn't count' about anything, because it does. Everything counts. Your energy counts, and your daily efforts in meeting the needs of your baby, or in your workplace, count too.

To make this crystal clear, it's likely that your ta-dah list might include: changing nappies, breastfeeding, making up bottles and feeding, washing up, tidying up, sterilising, doing laundry, making food, changing sheets, folding clothes, playing with your baby, getting your baby to sleep, life admin, booking appointments, texting someone back, commuting, meetings, tackling your inbox – you name it; write it down!

Ta-dah! List

When you get into bed, take a look at your list, add in anything you've forgotten, and really grant yourself a moment to take stock of everything you've packed into your awake hours. You will honestly be amazed and enlightened by how much goes unseen when you think you haven't done much, and hopefully this will start to help you reframe your own productivity.

I'd really recommend revisiting this activity (and A Mama's Worth on page 149) regularly – you could even try completing a ta-dah list every day for a week to get a real sense of what your new working hours entail. And remember that this is just the physical stuff. The emotional workload of motherhood is immense and deserves a serious amount of credit, so the next time you're feeling undervalued, remind yourself of this. Never has there been a job with efforts so unseen and effects so very valuable and, of course, deserving of and dependent on rest.

When you start completing regular ta-dah lists, I hope you'll start feeling like you've earned rest and reward yourself accordingly. Again, rest and relaxation doesn't have to present as grand gestures like spa days or massages. It could be something as simple as an early night or enjoying a hot cup of tea. Every time you complete your ta-dah list I want you to reward yourself with a moment that's just for you. Now there's an incentive if ever there was one.

RETURNING TO WORK

One of the biggest transitions that can happen in your baby's first year is the decision to return to work. Now obviously this is going to be different for everyone – some women will stay at home, some will

I make time to rest and nurture myself so that I can share myself with others

leave their old workplace and find something new, some will go back full-time and some flexibly. Some return to work after three months, some after six, nine, twelve months or more, and then there are those who are self-employed and don't have an official maternity leave at all. As you can see, there are so many possibilities and set-ups here, which means comparing ourselves to others is – yet again – a fruitless activity.

Going back to work after you've had your baby can feel like a really daunting prospect. You've been consumed with your little one for all these months – using a completely different part of your brain and personality than you're probably used to – and all of a sudden it's time for change again. I think one of the most difficult aspects of returning to work is the sense that you are making another transition when you've only just become comfortable with the last! It can feel really disorientating and you are certainly not alone in feeling anxious or unsure about what this change is going to look like. Similarly, you may be really excited to return to work, and that's fine too!

Looking forward to change or missing your job is no reflection on how much you love your baby, and as you're hopefully starting to understand, this is about finding *your* right, and *your* way.

Once you have decided on what your return to work is going to look like, try to give yourself lots of time to process your thoughts and feelings around this transition ahead of going back. Keep an open dialogue with your partner or support network, be honest and open about your feelings, and go easy on yourself. Here are some practical ideas you could consider:

Feel happy and confident with your childcare

We're going to look at childcare in more detail a little later on in this section (see page 217), but this is definitely something you want to spend lots of time getting right. Knowing that you are happy and trusting of who is looking after your little one will mean that you can navigate your own apprehensions and experience more attentively. Having peace of mind is paramount to you enjoying this new chapter, and you deserve that because you're doing something really brave.

Ease yourself back in gradually

If you are returning to work full-time, the idea of suddenly leaving your baby every day can sometimes feel upsetting or overwhelming, so maybe talk to your employer about using holiday to phase your return back to work. Easing yourself back in gently will enable you and your baby to make these big adjustments at a more relaxed pace, and learn your new routine together.

Set clear boundaries

Boundaries are a big deal in your motherhood journey, and we're going to be talking more about this a little later (see page 242). When you talk with your employer about returning to work, be really clear about what is expected of you and what you are/aren't willing to move on. We can all be flexible to a degree of course, but some things will feel essential to you and it's crucial that you communicate this so that you don't end up feeling resentful or guilty when you get back. For example, what's non-negotiable to you might be making sure you leave at a certain time, or whether you are happy to pick up emails at home etc. Working out these details before you go back means that everyone's expectations are aligned and you can focus all of your attention on being great at your job again.

Keep the dialogue open

For all the time we spend thinking about it, there's no knowing what returning to work will really feel like until it actually happens. Try to line up regular check-in chats with your employer and also your partner, support network and/or childcare so that you can all be honest and open about how things are going. This way, if something needs tweaking you can all work together for the best outcome, rather than waiting while tension builds. Remember that everyone involved in this chain is an adult, and conversation is the key to stronger connections all round.

Make time for yourself

One of the most difficult things about returning to work can be the sense of rushing around in order to squeeze everything in. Motherhood definitely feels like a full-time job emotionally, and you've now added more work on top of that. That's okay, but make sure you're taking the time you need to decompress between roles. Remember that you're likely to be feeling much more tired than you were before your baby came along – you're doing more than you ever have before and it's important to acknowledge and appreciate this for yourself. If you're commuting, you could try listening to the guided meditation that you'll get with this book (see page 7), doing some breath work or reading a book on your way home rather than continuing to check emails. This will help to reduce your stressor hormones and lift your endorphin levels so that you feel calm and at ease when you get home.

Don't be afraid to ask for help

As mothers we become adept at looking after everyone else, but let's not forget that we need help sometimes too. When we go through a big life transition (like having a baby or returning to work), it's important that we can lean on those who love us for emotional and practical support. Maybe you need help with some shopping, or just need a twenty-minute phone call with a friend to talk and offload. Don't underestimate the power of a conversation with someone juggling similar things to you. Maybe you have other mum friends who are returning to work at a similar time and could share the challenges by checking in with each other as you navigate the transition. Asking for what you need will lighten your load, and the people who love you will feel privileged that you've leant on them, I'm sure.

Regularly checking in with how you're feeling

While we might have quite a strong feeling of excitement or anxiety when we first return to work, it's likely that these will become more neutral as we settle into our new routine. In the beginning we can be on such a high state of alert that we're not necessarily focusing on the nuances of our new reality. Be proactive in checking in with yourself (try going back to those 'three simple questions' on page 174) about how you feel things are going and if there are any tweaks to be made.

Again, having these regular – scheduled if needs be – conversations as you go along rather than waiting until something is unbearable is a much healthier approach and one that everyone will benefit from.

I take control of what I can, and let go of what I can't

ACTIVITY

SAFE WORD

This activity is going to be a very handy part of your toolkit in the weeks, months and years ahead. It's one you can use on your own, or with other members of your household, and even with your children as they get a little older. The acronym we're going to focus on here is SAFE, and you're going to remember this whenever you need to reset or relax in times of transition or change.

Often when we face big life changes, we quickly feel overwhelmed and lose all of the calming and coping mechanisms we'd normally lean on. Having the word

SAFE embedded in your mind (much like you might have done when you affirmed 'I am safe' to yourself during transition in labour!) will help you to re-centre yourself quickly and effectively at a moment's notice.

Let's have a look at what it all means.

S slow down your breathing – notice the rise and fall of your breath without counting or controlling it. Just become aware of the rhythm of your stomach moving up and down, and connect with this gentle movement.

A affirm something valuable to yourself – in the instance of work, this could be something like 'I make decisions that feel right for me and my family' or 'I am always enough'.

F feel your feet on the ground – this is a brilliant way to mark the transition of leaving for work or returning home. Before you leave/arrive, take a moment to feel your feet firmly on the ground, and let this be reflected in your state of mind.

E exhale all worry – rather than carrying anxieties and worries around with you from place to place, recognise the importance of maintaining boundaries around your home and work life. Exhaling anything you don't need in this moment will help you leave work stuff at work, and home stuff at home, so that you can think clearly and be present where you're needed.

Try using this technique just around the idea of work to start with; so that could mean having conversations about returning to work, planning childcare, looking for work or starting back. Once you've become accustomed to using it here, you can use it in other areas of your life and reap that lovely sense of feeling clear-headed, present – and SAFE.

CHOICES, CHILDCARE AND CHANGE

Motherhood sometimes feels like a lifelong commitment to decision-making. What's the best thing? What's the right thing? Should I do this or that? What will the outcome be? It's easy to see why we can feel overwhelmed and intimidated by the weight of responsibility we carry for these beautiful babies. Just as we feel we've got one thing sorted, something else crops up and we're back to square one – weighing up our options and trying to turn down the outside noise, tune in to our instincts and make the decision that's best for our little family.

Childcare

Something that we'll often find ourselves thinking about in our baby's first year is childcare. It's not uncommon for people to think about this before their babies even arrive – especially those who have a predetermined end to maternity leave – but there's really no need to worry if you haven't considered your options this far in advance. I remember when I had my first son in 2010, lots of the mums I encountered were talking obsessively about nursery places and nanny-shares. These things hadn't even crossed my mind, and I suddenly felt panicked that I was three steps behind everyone else.

Motherhood can feel like this weird race at times: like you have to make the best decisions at the fastest pace. I know how easy it is to get caught up in this mindset, but I'm inviting you to sidestep it. What everyone else is doing doesn't dictate how you should make decisions, or what you should be thinking about.

Choosing childcare is a really personal thing, and it's okay to take your time, explore your options thoroughly, and slowly work out what will work for you and your family.

Given that it can feel like such an overwhelming topic, I want to give you a brief explanation of what your childcare options are. Much like when you considered where you were going to choose to have your baby, give each option some space to play out in your mind.

What would it look like?

How would it support your set-up?

How could it cause difficulties?

What does your gut say?

By weighing up the pros and cons of each option and then having considered conversations about each, you'll be able to make the right decision for you and your baby.

Nurseries

Nurseries will either be private or run by your local authority/council. Nurseries usually have the capacity to take babies from around three months old and until they are ready to start school. The size of nurseries will all vary, and many offer different educational approaches, for example Montessori or Steiner. Visit www.gov.uk/find-nursery-school-place to find out what your local area has to offer.

Childminders

Childminders are traditionally self-employed and usually take care of children in their own home, perhaps alongside their own child or a small number of other children. They are required to be Ofsted registered. If you go to www.gov.uk/find-registered-childminder, you'll be able to enter your postcode and then be given a list of registered childminders in your borough.

Nannies

A nanny is someone who is employed by a family to look after their child in the family home. Nanny-shares can also be a good option if you're looking to split the cost or only want childcare part-time. Nannies can be live-in or live-out, and you can decide what hours you require. Nannies will be registered on a Childcare Register and require a childcare qualification, DBS and first-aid certificate, but do not need to be Ofsted registered. Given that a nanny will be spending a large amount of time in your home, it's essential to find the right personal fit for your family.

Au pairs

An au pair is often a student from a different country who is here to better learn the language and experience living in the UK. An au pair will live with you as a temporary family member rather than an employee and is generally paid by way of a bedroom, meals and then a pre-agreed amount of pocket money per week/month. Generally speaking, au pairs do not have a childcare qualification and should not have sole charge of children under the age of two. You can visit www.aupairworld.com or www.aupair.com to find out more.

Other options

Some people will choose for a member of their family to look after their child, for instance a grandparent. This is obviously completely dependent on your personal set-up and is a much more informal childcare arrangement. There are other flexible and informal childcare set-ups available, such as pre-school playgroups, creches or children's centres. There is lots more information available at www.gov.uk/browse/childcare-parenting/childcare, including details of tax credits and childcare grants, which are well worth knowing your stuff on.

When exploring these options and trying to hone in on the type of childcare that might feel like the right fit for you and your family, consider some of these thinking points:

Why am I looking for childcare? For example, is it to enable a return to work, to give Mum some time off from childcare, or because you want your baby to socialise more?

What kind of environment does my baby thrive in? Remember that you are an expert on your baby! Do they love having one-to-one interactions or do they enjoy being among larger groups of children and other people?

When do we need it? Do you require childcare on a daily basis, once or twice a week, or on an ad-hoc basis?

How much does it cost? Finances are a big factor in choosing childcare, so it's a really good idea to work out what each option would cost based on the answers to the questions above.

What feels right for us? For example, would you feel happier taking your child somewhere else for childcare if you are going to be at home, or would you feel more comfortable with them staying in a home environment? Clue: There's no right or wrong answer!

It's worth carving out some space, too, to really reflect on how you feel about the prospect of childcare. It's all too easy for guilt to creep in on either side of the decision-making here: Am I depriving them of socialisation if I don't send them to nursery? Is it selfish of me to want time away from my baby? These are all things I've thought myself and heard hundreds of other mothers vocalise. By using the questions above as a starting point, you'll hopefully be able to calm some of these anxieties and consider a little bit of what everyone in the equation needs.

The same goes for when your little one actually starts a new arrangement. This new chapter can bring up a whole heap of complex emotions, and your best bet is to give them space to be felt, one at a time. Some babies seem completely unfazed by a new environment with new people, while others won't want to be let go of. Again, this is something that unfolds differently for everyone, and when you remember that there's no 'right' way for it to happen, you can nurture your baby (and yourself!) through each emotion of this big transition.

I make decisions that feel right for my family

If at all possible, it can be great to keep a clear diary around your little one entering a childcare setting. Not having the pressure of having to rush off to work, or to feel on edge during those early days, can be a really helpful way of navigating the ups and downs and overcoming any stumbling blocks together. Even a few days or a week to emotionally and physically hold space for this 'settling in' period will probably be something your future self thanks you for!

If and when you do choose to set up some childcare for your baby, remember that it's a big milestone and it's completely natural for it to feel daunting or overwhelming. There's no knowing how you're going to feel when your childcare gets started, but when we don't know what something's going to feel like, the best thing we can do is equip ourselves to calmly navigate unfamiliar territory.

Given that all of motherhood is *largely* unfamiliar territory, you're probably already way better at this than you think, but let's recap on some tips and tricks to reaffirm your capabilities and coping mechanisms. There's also an activity I'm going to introduce you to shortly that has become my go-to exercise when I'm trying to reconcile conflicting thoughts or feelings. It's well worth a try because I think you'll like it, too! Hop on over to the Tidy Drawer Challenge on page 224 if you want to get stuck in.

1. ***Focus on your breath***
   Remember that your breath holds the power to short-circuit our stressor responses and stop adrenaline in its tracks. When we regulate our breathing and quieten our mind, we are better equipped to deal with difficult feelings or anxiety as they arise. Try the Calm Breath on page 33, the Take Five technique on page 143 or the Breather Branches on page 42.

2. *Write down your worries*
   Getting our fears and anxieties out of our mind and down onto paper can offer up a welcome opportunity to see and process them in a more calm and rational way. Remember that it's often when we get into bed at night that our mind starts whirring with all of these thoughts, so keep a little notebook by the side of your bed and do a quick brain audit before you go to sleep. Writing or journaling also gives us an opportunity to see what particular elements of a fear or worry we're most affected by, rather than it just feeling huge and overwhelming.

3. *Look for the positives*
   Every single challenge holds within it a blessing of some kind, and when we are able to quieten our minds (see points 1 and 2) we create space for these to surface. If you're feeling anxious about your little one starting nursery for instance, try writing down all the positive things that could come from it. It's normal to feel worried or unsure about how something like this is going to unfold, but by focusing on the positives we become more open to receiving them.

ACTIVITY

THE TIDY DRAWER CHALLENGE

Okay, stick with me. I know what you're thinking, but this is honestly my most effective go-to technique when I am feeling uncertain or anxious about a particular event or course of action.

One of the biggest adjustments I think we make as mothers is trying to get comfortable with having less control and less organisation in our homes. Our cultural norms are set up around order, routine and structure, and when this tiny person turns up with no idea about those things, it can make many elements of our life suddenly feel less calm or controllable. Add to that the physical chaos that little people often create, and it's no wonder that we frequently feel frazzled and less equipped to process our experiences, feelings and challenges with the same level of clarity we may have done before.

In this activity, you're going to tidy or organise one drawer or cupboard in your house, while processing something you feel worried or conflicted about. So let's say that's childcare, or returning to work, seeing as they're the things we've just been talking about.

1. First of all, take everything out of this drawer or cupboard. Start with something simple like babygros, socks or make-up so that it's not going to take you all afternoon to put things back in order.
2. As you're taking items out of the drawer, think about what's informing your worry or concern. Try saying the worry out loud as you take an item out.
3. When everything is out of the drawer, have a look at what you've got in front of you. Some of the things you'll want to throw/pack/give away, whereas some of them you'll want to keep.
4. Assign the worries that are out of your control to the items you are not putting back in the drawer. Set them aside.
5. Assign the thoughts that you can manage or sit with to the items you're going to put back in the drawer. As you fold each item and put it back, connect with the idea that you have tidied your thoughts and they can sit peacefully in your mind for a time where you might need them.

And that's it – a tidier drawer, more organised thoughts and a less overwhelming state of mind! Have a go at doing this whenever your mind is feeling cluttered. I guarantee you'll feel better for it – and you'll have an easier time finding your favourite pair of socks tomorrow, too.

RECONNECTING WITH YOUR PARTNER

We know only too well how our baby's needs are constant and demanding to begin with, but keep in mind that the energy that's been taken out of your relationship over these months needs to be put back in further down the line. Our primal instincts and energies carry us through those early days, but as our baby grows and their needs become more predictable, we can start to redirect some of this attention back to ourselves and our loved ones, and now can be a great time to really embrace doing this.

One of the biggest strains on any relationship in the first year of parenthood is sleep deprivation (don't forget to memorise my all-important tips for coping with sleep deprivation on page 101). Having a baby is like a 24-hour job to share *on top of* your other jobs. It's physical and it's emotional. It's huge, and it creates a very immediate sense of pressure and strain, even in the strongest relationships. It's easy to become disconnected during your baby's first year (and even beyond that) – to compete rather than connect, and to become resentful and angry if you feel your efforts (in whatever capacity) aren't being appreciated. This can manifest in different ways as your children grow, because parenting is naturally consuming and it does create a forever-shift in our role as partners, so having tools for reconnecting along the way is essential. Ultimately, I think we all just want someone to say 'you're doing such a good job and I value you', and actually when we hear this, we immediately feel more relaxed, more at ease, and better connected. Let's look at how we can make this more achievable when the odds are stacked against us.

Experiencing breakdowns in communication when you've had a baby is inevitable. Your energy and resources are being more thinly spread, you have less time to nurture your own needs (let alone the needs of another adult) and your loving energy is being tirelessly diverted to your baby. While this might seem daunting, I'm inviting you now to see it from another, more positive angle: that every disconnection or disagreement offers an opportunity to repair and reconnect.

Think about it. Even when there isn't a baby in the equation, it's impossible to be attentive, agreeable and available to your partner all of the time. We all have flaws, we all miscommunicate, we all say mean things sometimes. We all have worries and pressures that we are trying to navigate, and this can add strain to our relationships, baby or not! We disagree, argue and withdraw – these are normal reactions to pain and suffering. What matters is how we deal with these fluctuations.

What matters is our commitment to repair,
a willingness to improve our interactions,
and the courage to reach out for reconnection.

Earlier on in the book we looked at how to nurture your relationship in the very early days of parenthood, but given that this is a long game with ever-changing obstacles, we need to keep working at it and refreshing our approach to reconnection. In this activity I am inviting both you and your partner to be more considered in how you communicate. I am inviting you to take responsibility for your emotional contributions to conflict and to be proactive in the process of reconnecting. I am inviting you to recognise that the value of your relationship is *always* more important than any problem it faces.

ACTIVITY

RECOGNITION AND RECONNECTION

For this to be effective, you both need to identify how you react when you are feeling scared, defensive or angry. Do you withdraw? Do you attack? Do you sulk? Do you shout? Do you martyr yourself? Do you shame? Do you ignore? When you can acknowledge your conflict reflexes, you can work out a more compassionate approach to replace it with. Let me give you some examples.

You feel criticised.

Your conflict reflex is to retaliate with an attack or criticism.

Rather than retaliating, what happens if you say, 'I feel criticised and it makes me feel like retaliating. Can you rephrase what you're saying in a softer way?'

You don't feel like you get enough help.

Your conflict reflex is to attack by shaming your partner's lack of contribution.

Rather than shaming, what happens if you say, 'I'm feeling overwhelmed, please can you help me?'

You and your partner have opposing opinions over something.

Your conflict reflex is to dig your heels in and become obstinate.

Rather than withdrawing and facing a stand-off, what happens if you say, 'Let's take turns to listen to each other and find our common ground.'?

The key to this becoming an effective way to strengthen how you communicate is that you are both on board with trying. It's not always going to go right, and there will still be disagreements and disconnections. This activity invites you to be aware of your contributions in a crisis, though, and to find kinder, more connected ways to reach solutions.

As soon as you start feeling the benefits of reconnection, you'll be spurred on to make a conscious effort in developing this skill and it will become easier *and* more effective. Use the space overleaf to identify your conflict reflexes, and also to write down instances where you've managed to reconnect. The more frequently you log these, the better!

Try to remember that it is absolutely inevitable that your relationship will come under strain when you have a baby. How strain manifests will vary from couple to couple, but it might include things like having less sex, not talking as much, spending less time together, less laughter, not making as much effort for each other, one or both of you having a shorter fuse, and so on. All of these things are completely normal, and it doesn't mean your relationship is doomed.

While the first chunk of life with your baby is likely to feel like it's all hands on deck, as the months and years go on our roles can often take more clear and divided paths. Perhaps one person is staying at home more while the other works, perhaps you split childcare and work equally; this can all potentially change, and more than once, as life goes on. Maybe you will enlist childcare, or maybe switch roles. Having the tools to weather these logistical storms to find your own flow and equilibrium will stand you in great stead for the onward journey, so let's continue to think about how we can do that, and keep tooling up!

Today I let love lead me

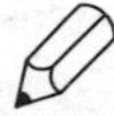

ACTIVITY

GRATITUDE EXCHANGE

The older your little one gets, the more pockets of time and space you'll start to find for inviting back parts of your pre-baby reality. We've already talked about this in terms of our own identity on pages 117, 133 and 199, but we can apply it to our relationships – and friendships – too.

If you think back to the beginning of your relationship, I bet you'll be able to recall kind things you did for each other. If one of you made dinner, organised a date, or sent a kind and loving text message, it was probably really well received and appreciated. The reality of life with little ones means that grand gestures can be difficult, but the kindness of small gestures on a daily basis can form the glue that holds your bond tight and together, and that's where this gratitude exchange comes in.

Every single day, from now, I want you to end the day by telling the other person one thing you're grateful to them for. Even if you're tired, have had an argument or aren't physically together (maybe one of you is away for work), making this a daily part of your routine will help you to both feel valued and loved, and to more easily mend disconnections when they inevitably arise.

When considering what you're grateful to your partner for, keep it simple. Remember that we're not looking for grand gestures, we're looking for the small things that might otherwise go unseen. So it could be: feeding baby or making up a bottle in the night; making the bed; running the other a bath; cooking dinner; picking up essentials; taking out the bins; going to work for the family. Say it out loud and be open to receiving this gratitude, too. Acknowledging and appreciating the seemingly mundane builds the foundations for your gratitude and love for one another to flourish in even bigger ways.

To keep you on track, use the space opposite to write down what your partner has said they're grateful to you for every day for a week, so that when you're feeling undervalued, you can look back and remind yourself otherwise.

Make time for your physical relationship as well. With a newborn stuck to our bodies in one way or another for the first few months, not to mention the tiredness that kicks in from the off, it's easy to understand how the physical aspects of our partnerships can get overlooked. The attention we give to each other falls to the bottom of the pile when we have other things that are so immediately demanding, but now's the time to pull it back up and give it some space on stage.

Your sex life might look pretty different to how it did in your pre-baby days, but don't be disheartened. Intimacy takes so many forms, and by focusing on strengthening these foundations, your sex life will start getting topped up with the energy and attention it might need. Now

Monday

Tuesday

Wednesday

Thursday

Friday

Saturday

Sunday

you may well be one of these couples that jumps straight back into an exciting sex life in the weeks or months following your baby's birth and that's great, but it's just as normal (and probably more common) for that not to happen quite so quickly.

Let's think about some ways you can introduce physical love and intimacy back into your relationship, one step at a time.

Talk to your partner. Yes, it sounds obvious but talking about how you're feeling is key here. None of us want to reach the point where this becomes the elephant in the room, and even saying something like 'do you think we'll ever have sex again?!' can break the ice and offer a gentle way back in to exploring things more.

Reminisce about the things you used to enjoy. Again, this is all based on the connectedness of conversation, but reflecting on fun and intimate times you've shared might provide just the inspiration and motivation you need to start revisiting things you enjoy.

Touch each other, and I mean in the simplest of ways. Hold hands when you're out or pushing the buggy, have a cuddle when you get into bed at night, or stroke each other's head/arms/feet while you're watching TV in the evening. Remember that stroking or gentle touching stimulates the nerve endings on our skin and makes the body produce endorphins and oxytocin – our hormones of love and happiness!

Compliment each other whenever you can. Receiving compliments boosts our endorphin levels and we naturally feel more relaxed and ready to connect. This could be as simple as 'I love the way you smell' or 'you always make me laugh and I love that' or 'you cook the best curry!' – again it doesn't have to be too try-hard, it's more about noticing the day-to-day stuff that you might otherwise take for granted.

Be kind and gentle with each other, and remember that this is part of your journey – the downs as well as the ups. Every time you navigate a challenging set of circumstances, you are building your resilience and working out your stride as a team.

This is the way to do it. It's not always going to feel great, but learning to hold each other tight in the trickier times will help you relish the better ones even more, and if you look out for it, there is so much joy to be shared on this ride called parenting.

LIFE AS A SOLO PARENT

If you are on this journey as a solo parent, it's just as important (maybe even more so) to know that you are never alone. Single-parent families are more common than ever, and finding ways to feel supported and valued in your journey as a mother is really crucial. Whether you're a solo parent by choice or circumstance, it can be hard to juggle the challenges of parenthood when we're managing the responsibility alone, and don't have someone on tap to tell us we're doing a great job.

The physical and emotional responsibilities go way beyond looking after your baby, and you want to feel fully equipped and supported in raising your child in the years to come, however that may unfold. The most valuable (and underrated) element of being an effective parent (whether that's a co-parent or a solo parent) is looking after yourself. Having an outlet for how you feel and giving yourself permission to feel anxious or overwhelmed at times is really important. Learning to identify these feelings will mean you can ask for support when you need it, and equip yourself with some coping mechanisms to make the more challenging times that little bit easier.

It may be that you are well supported by family and friends, or by a group of other parents. These people may prove to be an incredible source of love and support for you when you need it most, and make life easier by giving you practical or logistical support too. It may be though that you are completely alone and don't have a network to fall back on. If this is the case then I would really recommend reaching out to local or national organisations or charities who can support you with all manner of things, from finances to more hands-on support.

Practical support tips for solo parents

A step ahead: When you're one-on-one with your baby all the time, it can be really helpful to stay organised and ahead of yourself. This doesn't require any kind of life overhaul, but rather simple things like getting out what you/your baby need for the next morning the night before, or batch-cooking rather than having to do it every night.

Create a routine: When you haven't got someone to juggle the load with, routine and a gentle structure to your days can provide the support you might feel like you're sometimes lacking. Knowing when you're going to cook, when you're going to do chores and when you're going to relax and have some downtime means it's all more likely to happen and feel less overwhelming.

Find childcare that works: Traditional childcare isn't going to be a chosen or accessible option for everyone, but as your baby gets older, there may be ways that you can source some childcare that suits your set-up. If you can find a qualified caregiver by way of a nursery, nanny or childminder then brilliant, but you can come at this from a more creative angle, too. If you can find a trustworthy babysitter, maybe they could sit and play with your baby for a few hours while you do something for yourself at home. If you know other solo parents or have a great network of mum friends, see if you can take it in turns to help each other out. It can be amazing just to have that mental breather, even if it's only every so often (and also see Choices, Childcare and Change on page 217).

Accept and ask for help when you need it: Whether you need help with your finances or logistical support with older children, don't be afraid to seek it out and accept it. Have a look for online or social support groups for solo parents where there's bound to be access to more practical and emotional support, or contact local charities or organisations who can help you with more specific concerns. Getting your finances in order can relieve a huge amount of pressure, especially when there is only one of you carrying the weight, and lots of networks or organisations specialise in exactly this.

Emotional support tips for solo parents

Ditch the guilt: Don't compare yourself to anyone who has twice the number of hands on deck. You are doing your best and that is enough. It's more than enough actually. If your baby is loved and safe then you are absolutely excelling at this motherhood lark and don't forget it! If social media or mum groups are making you doubt yourself or feel guilty, take a temporary step away from them and see if you feel better. Noticing who or what your energy increases and decreases around can be a great gauge for adjusting anything that negatively impacts your energy or self-esteem.

Make time for yourself: In the early days you may well be using every quiet moment to sleep, frantically shower or recoup your precious energy, but as your baby gets older and their routine becomes a little more predictable, start setting aside regular pockets of time to top up your tank. Learn a skill you've always wanted to (this could be in-person classes or online) or join a book club (check out the All The Things I Love exercise on page 199 for more inspiration!). Having access to adult company and conversation can be really important for connecting with your identity and interests again. The older your baby gets, the easier this becomes, so hang on in there – you're doing GREAT!

Use affirmations: When there are two of you sharing the load of parenting it can be easier to give each other that emotional boost when it's needed most; when you're on your own it's something that can require a bit more conscious effort. Affirmations offer a really easy and effective way of doing this. If you're doubting yourself or having a wobble, turn that worry or fear into a confident, positive statement of the opposite. For example 'I am everything my child needs' or 'I am a strong, capable mother'. You can write these down for yourself and repeat them aloud as often as you can!

Compliments and gratitude: Following on from the above, be the loving voice your mother heart needs sometimes. There are positive affirmations sprinkled throughout this book, so if some of them really speak to you, try writing them down to think upon more regularly. It may just help you to speak more kindly to yourself, express your gratitude to yourself and acknowledge every single thing you accomplish.

I am exactly what my child needs

BOUNDARIES

If we want to develop healthy, safe and loving relationships with our children, this must be what we're modelling in our immediate relationships. From the youngest age, our children observe and digest all sorts of behavioural cues that become their pillars for normality. The most wonderful thing about becoming a parent is that we have the chance to shape someone's world, but with this comes a responsibility to observe and adjust our own.

Having a baby can bring up a lot of emotions about your own childhood. It can shape what kind of parent you want to be, from traditions to discipline and everything in between. Some of us will want to recreate everything our parents did, while others will want to do the polar opposite, but let's imagine there's space for something in the middle once we've set our boundaries (and this is something you can also consider and explore in more detail with your Motherhood Mood Board on page 179).

How you decide to raise your children sits with you and you alone. I'm not here to tell you how to do that. What I'm aiming to do is give you the confidence to trust your instincts and make the decisions that feel right for you and your family along the way, just like we talked about when we looked at strengthening our intuition muscle on page 168. I also want you to feel calm and unafraid when you need to change direction, or tweak something that doesn't feel like it's the right fit for your little unit.

What we're working towards here is remaining active participants in our lives and those of our children. By considering what our options are and making informed choices, we can relax and enjoy the journey in a much more empowering and liberating way, free from the shackles of other people's opinions, and, as such, liberate our children to do the same.

As we become better and braver at identifying our beliefs, setting our boundaries and of course communicating them to others, this gets easier and becomes more like an innate reflex than a conscious effort.

There are likely to be times in your parental journey (now and well into the years to come!) where you'll need to assert yourself and communicate what you are and are not happy with. This sounds easier to do than it often is in reality, since many of us are conditioned people-pleasers. It can take a little unlearning and relearning along the way. Before we can communicate well with others, we need to learn to listen to and respond to ourselves – to notice how we feel and what we really want, as opposed to what we think we should do or how we should react. The next exercise is going to help with this.

ACTIVITY

EMBRACING THE POWER OF YES AND NO

How often do we find ourselves saying yes when we really want to say no? I haven't met many people who can't relate to that, and I guess it's because we've been conditioned to people-please from a young age.

Often because of our own upbringings, we are afraid to disappoint people or we feel anxious about conflict, and so we prioritise other people's experiences ahead of our own; but this can often lead to feelings of anger and resentment that bubble away under the surface until we can't take it any more and explode. This could manifest as a big argument or blow-up, or as a drip-drip of agitation directed towards those closest to us. To prevent this from happening, it's really important that we learn *when* to say yes and *how* to say no.

In this activity, I'm going to give you three brilliant tips for practising this, and I'm inviting you to exercise your yes and no muscles. The stronger these muscles get, the easier it will become to create and maintain boundaries not only for yourself, but for your little ones too, and that's when you can really start to enjoy motherhood, your way.

Learn to say yes to yourself

While you might be well versed in dishing out yeses here, there and everywhere, how often do you say yes to yourself? How often do you talk yourself out of deserving or needing something, like rest, sleep or pleasure? The first part of this activity is finding three opportunities to say yes to yourself. After all, if we want our children to have the confidence and freedom to serve themselves, we have to start by modelling it for them. Pay attention to this idea over the next week or so, and write those three opportunities down overleaf as and when they appear.

The better we get at saying yes to ourselves, the more thoughtfully we can consider offering it out to others. When we've given ourselves what we really need, we have a more realistic view of our reserves and capacity, and this means we're more likely to say yes without overstretching ourselves.

Pause, breathe, think

The next time someone asks something of you, try not giving an answer straight away. Giving yourself time to consider your resources means you're more able to make a decision that reflects how you really feel. Ask for a bit of time to get back to them, or say you'd like a bit of time to think it over. I always feel calmer when I make decisions in my own time rather than react on the spot. This is a bit like what we practise in labour – making informed decisions calmly and slowly.

Try bringing the request or what's been asked of you to mind and then hold it there. Take three nice Calm Breaths (see page 33) and then note how you feel about the proposition. Clearing your mind and sitting with your thoughts and feelings will help you to tune in to your intuition (see page 168), and make the decision that really feels right for you. It might be a struggle at first, but the more you exercise it, the easier it gets.

Again, use the space on the opposite page to work out your thoughts the next time something's asked of you.

Keep it simple/resist the urge to explain

When you are saying no, try to resist the urge to explain or make someone feel better. We can be polite and assertive at the same time – they are not mutually exclusive, and the only way to really accept that is to try it and realise nothing terrible happens as a consequence of you politely saying 'no' or 'no thank you'.

If this feels too difficult when you're getting started, you could precede no with 'I feel really appreciative that you've chosen to ask me that' so that you can acknowledge with kindness your choice to say no this time. Use the space on the opposite page to note down occasions where you've said no, and jot down, draw or doodle about the way it felt.

Don't worry if this exercise feels really difficult or uncomfortable at first. Lots of us will find that making conscious yes and no choices doesn't come easily, but a lot of this is about realising that nothing terrible happens when we assert ourselves. And this is just the beginning. Learning how to say yes and no is a very simple step towards understanding our own boundaries, and how that affects our relationships with those around us.

> Clear, kind and consistent boundaries are vital to healthy, respectful relationships, and this is a brilliant skill to not only develop as mothers, but to model for our children.

The more attention we can give to bringing clarity in the way we communicate, the fewer opportunities there are for emotional conflict and confusion. We are all responsible for our own happiness, and this starts with showing ourselves very basic levels of honesty and expressing them outwards.

Okay, so I think you'll probably agree that we've been exploring some trickier thought processes here, and doing some of the more emotional unpacking that's par for the parental course, so let's take some time now to really celebrate and acknowledge how much deep and potentially difficult work we're doing. Have a go at the really wonderful exercise on the next page – it might be my favourite activity in the whole book!

We've talked a lot about our invisible workload as mums, haven't we? You are feeding, cleaning, responding, loving, shushing, rocking, emotionally computing... and the list goes on (and on), but they are things that often go unseen. I'm here to remind you – again! – that your work is absolutely amazing. Yes, it can still sometimes feel horribly relentless and exhausting at times, but giving yourself the love and credit you deserve will go a long way in spurring you on to enjoy this ride, your way. This activity is going to help you acknowledge all your great work, and give you an ongoing appraisal!

ACTIVITY

LOVE NOTES TO YOURSELF

Find an empty jar, and label it 'love notes to myself'. You are going to fill it with just that. Every single day, I want you to write something and put it in that jar. As the name says, we are not talking here about long letters; they just need to be little notes jotted down from you to you, to remind yourself what an awesome job you're doing. If you're not in the habit of being loving towards yourself, then here are some ideas to get you started:

'You are brilliant at staying calm, even when it's not easy. You rock!'

'I know you're really tired, but you are doing an amazing job and you are enough.'

'Your baby loves you so much, and feels so safe with you.'

'Remember that it's okay to change plans, say no, and prioritise yourself. Motherhood can be really challenging and you deserve to show yourself that kindness.'

You can even invite your partner or friends to contribute too. Every time you're feeling the strain, or just a bit flat, go to your jar and pick out a love note for yourself. If you have children already, you can even encourage everyone in your household to make one and watch the magic, confidence and compassion explode!

YOUR BABY

A lot starts happening in our baby's little world when they get to the six-month mark and beyond. You may well have started introducing solid foods, they could be starting to sit up or show efforts to crawl, and maybe, ***maybe***, they're starting to sleep for slightly longer or more predictable periods of time.

From an attachment perspective, your baby continues to develop that discriminate preference for their primary caregiver, so in the moments you feel that sense of pressure or overwhelm at how much your baby needs from you, try to remember that it's because they think you're the most awesome, reliable and trustworthy person on the planet! In order to create the space to enjoy that, let's look at some of the ways you can strengthen your connection with your baby, how you can support and nurture their development, and how you can bond with each other in your very own, unique ways.

HELPING YOUR BABY TO THRIVE

On every step of your motherhood journey, remember that no one knows your baby better than you. You are an expert in your baby, and you always, always know best when it comes to their happiness and well-being. Your baby is going to reach common milestones at their own, perfect pace. Obsessing over these and comparing their accomplishments to others can really suck the joy out of watching them. Remember, too, that their developments aren't always visible. They are constantly evolving and learning, and growing emotionally as well as physically. Celebrate the uniqueness of what they are doing – keep a little log of the lovely things you notice about them, and don't give too much thought to what they're yet to figure out.

Language

Your baby won't be talking just yet, but don't let that fool you into thinking language isn't a huge part of their life. They are likely to start making more repetitive sounds now (like da-da or ga-ga) and you can nurture this new skill in two great ways. First of all, try repeating the sounds your baby makes. Make the same sound back to them, wait, and see if they do it again. By doing this you are teaching them about the rhythm of a conversation – a skill they will continue to observe and process over the coming months. Another way to support and nurture their linguistic development is to talk to them about what you're doing, or find the words to describe their experience for them. For example, 'I think you're thirsty aren't you?' or 'I can see you feel sad when we have to stop playing.' The more we talk, the more they hear and learn and the more they feel safe. These skills all contribute to those feelings of attachment, security and connectedness. This is just one example of the huge value in your everyday work.

Play

The older your baby gets, the more fun and interactive your playtimes become. We've already talked about the power of imitation and copying (see page 129), and you may continue to notice that your baby copies physical movements you make. This is a form of communication and connection, and I'd encourage you to reciprocate. A game like peek-a-boo really comes into its own around this age, and is a great way to reassure babies who might be starting to experience separation anxiety. Earlier on, I suggested doing this in a very simple way – hiding behind a piece of fabric for example – but as your baby gets older you can evolve this. Hiding and then reappearing reassures your baby that you're still there, even when he can't see you. Isn't that a wonderful thing to learn?

Routine

Now that your baby is growing, your days will probably feature a bit more familiarity and structure, which can definitely be used to your advantage in terms of creating that sense of safety and security with your little one. While I've talked about the potential stumbling blocks of trying to enforce a routine too early on (see pages 22 and 100), identifying and upholding natural rhythms that act as anchors throughout your day can be super-helpful and beneficial at this point. For example, finding a way to help your baby wind down when it's getting close to bedtime can be really useful. Maybe that's a bath, watching a particular programme or reading a certain story, having a cuddle, or enjoying their milk with you – whatever these little hallmarks look like, they can become an easy way for your baby to identify that bedtime is coming and respond positively to this familiar routine of some quality, loving moments with you.

Having these little practices or rituals in place also means that if you go away with your baby, or if someone else looks after them, there are ways to keep consistency and calmness on the agenda amid unavoidable changes. I always sang my little one the same song before bed, and after a while I started to feel his body physically relax, as if he was surrendering to bedtime in the most trusting and familiar way.

You can use these types of anchors at any time of day and adapt them as your baby gets older. With my littlest now a toddler, he knows that when we go out we sit on the step to put our shoes on, and it also means that as it becomes relevant and age-appropriate, they can start to assert some autonomy over their participation, which is amazing.

Remember that every baby will respond differently and at varied paces to routine, and that routine doesn't just mean sleep. Some will fall into recognisable rhythms in a heartbeat, whereas others require a little more trial and error and lots of tweaking along the way. Again, there's no right or wrong way of introducing this kind of thing – identify what would be useful and complementary to your family, and create some ideas about how you could implement simple, loving structures throughout your day. Also remember that some days this will inevitably all go out of the window, and that's okay too!

We all have our off days, babies included, so remember that each day brings us an opportunity to try again. Be patient with yourself and don't be afraid to change direction if something doesn't feel quite right for you. Every family is different.

This feels like a good time to say that the first year of being a parent (and, of course, beyond) can bring up many emotions that feel overwhelming, disorientating and exhausting. I'd love to say that this subsides, but rather I think you just get used to living alongside it. Whether it's a change in your family dynamics, a child starting school, another baby or other momentous changes, the feelings you process as a parent can feel fast and furious. Your breathing techniques are always on hand in these moments of emotional madness, but let's look at some more ways to get back to basics when you need it most.

SLOWING DOWN AND RECONNECTING

What if it suddenly feels like life is becoming very fast-paced again? Maybe you're returning to work, or are taking on more responsibilities elsewhere. Maybe your partner is working longer hours or you have lots going on with other children. It's really important that you know how to check in with yourself and that you are able to slow down and reconnect when you need it most. Noticing your triggers is key here. How do you feel when things are getting too much? Do you have trouble sleeping? Do you have a shorter fuse? Feel snappy with your partner? Cry more? Eat more sugar? Becoming aware of your stress-signposts can make way for more awareness in addressing this stress and taking time to rest and reset.

In this next activity, I want to give you the opportunity to press pause when everything's feeling a bit much, and take things right back to the early days when life was slow and simple. There is nothing to say we have to keep ploughing on when we're feeling exhausted and depleted.

Productivity and presenteeism are social constructs, and while it might not always be realistic, we *can* choose to hop off every so often. Pressing pause like this can give us the opportunity to gather our thoughts and resources, regroup, and re-emerge feeling calmer and more energised.

It's also incredibly liberating to realise that nothing terrible happens when you hunker down for a couple of days. The world keeps spinning and you can hop back on when you're ready.

Today I will slow down and try not to rush

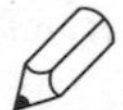

ACTIVITY

ENJOYING A BELATED BABY BUBBLE

A belated baby bubble simply means recreating a calm, slow and nurturing space a little further down the line. Think of it as a holiday at home, where you can pull up the drawbridge from the outside world and retreat back into your little nest. Clear your diary for a few days or a week – and that means making no commitments whatsoever – and dedicate your time purely to looking after yourself and connecting with your baby. You might want to consider some or all of these things:

- If you have one, can you include your partner so that you can share the workload of your baby but also savour in the joy of going slow together? If getting the time off work isn't a possibility, maybe set your belated baby bubble up as a long weekend instead. This isn't one-size-fits-all; it's about making the time work for you.
- If you have older children, see if you can plan in advance and arrange a playdate or two, so that you can max out the bubble days.
- Do some batch-cooking for the freezer in advance of your bubble, or stock up on some pre-cooked meals

that you can freeze. It can also be a nice opportunity to get in a few bars of your favourite chocolate (a great endorphin-booster!) or other indulgent treat. This is your time to truly reward yourself for all the amazing work you've been doing! Plus, not having to worry about cooking will free up time to enjoy those cuddles with your baby and really rest.

- Book an at-home massage, or have an afternoon bath with your favourite oils and candles. You want to think of this as a time for giving back to your body – it's worked so hard and brilliantly, and continues to. The more relaxed and at ease you are, the more readily available you'll feel for your baby.
- Watch a movie in bed while cuddling your baby. This sounds so simple, but I found it to be such a good way to relax in your baby bubble. It also means you can get cosy and enjoy lots of endorphin-boosting skin-to-skin with your little one. Watching a great film always stops my mind thinking about the million things I have going on – a bit of a creative escape I guess – but in those first few months with baby, I could never ever stay awake long enough in the evening to watch one!

Remember that these are just my ideas for what makes a perfect baby bubble; everyone has their own preferences when it comes to rest, relaxation and reconnection with your little one, so don't be afraid to tailor yours to your own heart and soul. The aim is to spend a couple of days looking after yourself, bonding with your baby, and not worrying about the world outside of your door for a little pocket of time. It rests your mind, recharges your body, and can be the perfect way to reset and realign for your onward journey.

This is one of those great activities that you can adapt as time goes on and depending on what you feel you need, and it certainly doesn't have to be a one-off either! Even now, if I'm feeling depleted, tired or run-down, I know it will only get worse if I don't address it. I look for a free-ish day that week, cancel any plans, ask a friend to have my bigger boy after school, and take it super-easy – eating good food, taking a long bath and catching up on my favourite series while Cosmo sleeps. Sometimes it only takes one day or even an afternoon of self-care to press the reset button, and I would highly encourage you to give it a go! It always makes me feel like a better mother because I inevitably become less stressed and more emotionally available to my children, which is a positive thing for everyone!

OVERCOMING OVERWHELM

A really useful technique for overcoming overwhelm when it comes to our responsibilities (or the choices we have to make) as mothers is to reframe how we view this mental load. In this activity, we're going to try tweaking the way we think about what is expected or asked of us, and turning it from a chore into a treat.

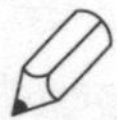

ACTIVITY

PRIVILEGE PERSPECTIVE

To reframe how we think of our responsibilities, we're simply going to replace the phrase *have to* with *get to*. For example, the next time you get up to see to your baby at three o'clock in the morning and you think 'I *have to* get up,' try mentally rephrasing it with 'I *get to* get up'. This isn't about ignoring that things feel hard sometimes, but rather creating mental shifts that help us see something that we'll inevitably do anyway as a privilege.

There are some more examples below, but use the space to write down your own observations and switches, too.

I have to wash all of these sleepsuits or *I get to wash all of these sleepsuits*

I have to hold her all day or *I get to hold her all day*

I have to do bath time or I get to do bath time

I have to make packed lunches every day or I get to feed my children every day

This activity gets better and better the older your child gets. I still try to do it when I'm running around like a taxi service for my eldest, or cooking family meals. Acknowledging the joy and privilege in what I'm providing can really help to shift my perspective, and can (more often than not!) turn resentment into gratitude in a matter of moments.

NAVIGATING THE UNEXPECTED

When you're a mum, every time you feel you've mastered something you'll be surprised or caught off guard by something new and unexpected. It can feel like an ongoing apprenticeship at times, can't it? This can be a really *really* difficult thing to get your head around, because we've never had to deal with something so unpredictable before.

I wish I could say this gets easier but I don't think it does. What happens is that you get better at navigating it, and that, I promise you, is true. Already you will be dealing with things so much more calmly and easily than you might have done six or more months ago. Maybe it doesn't always feel that way, but I bet it's true. In the early days, I'm sure that every noise or grumbling your baby made had you on high alert. Now you take these things in your stride, trusting that growing instinct and relying confidently upon your deep-rooted maternal wisdom that materialises more as each day passes. You know what's normal for your baby, you're more closely aligned to your feelings and beliefs about the type of mother you're becoming, and you're learning to control the things you can and let go of the things you can't.

As you continue to learn and grow, I want to share with you a wonderful technique that will help to keep you feeling grounded, confident and well equipped in navigating anything that life throws your way – and this can go way beyond being baby-related. We all know that life happens, and not always in a way we've envisaged. Work, friendships, relationships, family – all of these things can throw up their curveballs, and facing these challenges with a toolkit of self-belief and resilience will better equip you to find your way through them. This is one to take some time over and to slowly enjoy building over a few days, weeks or even months. It's your Tree of Self-Belief. Let me explain.

ACTIVITY

THE TREE OF SELF-BELIEF

On the page opposite you'll see a sound and solid tree. Blossoming from it are lots of blank leaves, and these are going to become hosts to all of your skills and coping strategies, which are what form your tree of self-belief.

Over the coming days and weeks, start identifying your personal strengths (this can include you as a mother, lover, friend, daughter, colleague – all the layers of your identity!), your coping skills and strategies, and the supportive people, places or things that help get you through difficult or unfamiliar territory.

Write each of these things onto a blank leaf. They could include all manner of things: reading, exercise, being kind, a sense of humour, creativity, bed, sleep, communication, nature, a good friend, and so on. You can even add more leaves onto the tree, or draw a new (bigger!) one on a separate piece of paper, and keep it somewhere helpful.

Whenever you're feeling overwhelmed or ill-equipped to deal with what life is putting in front of you, bring yourself to your tree and muse upon your blossoming

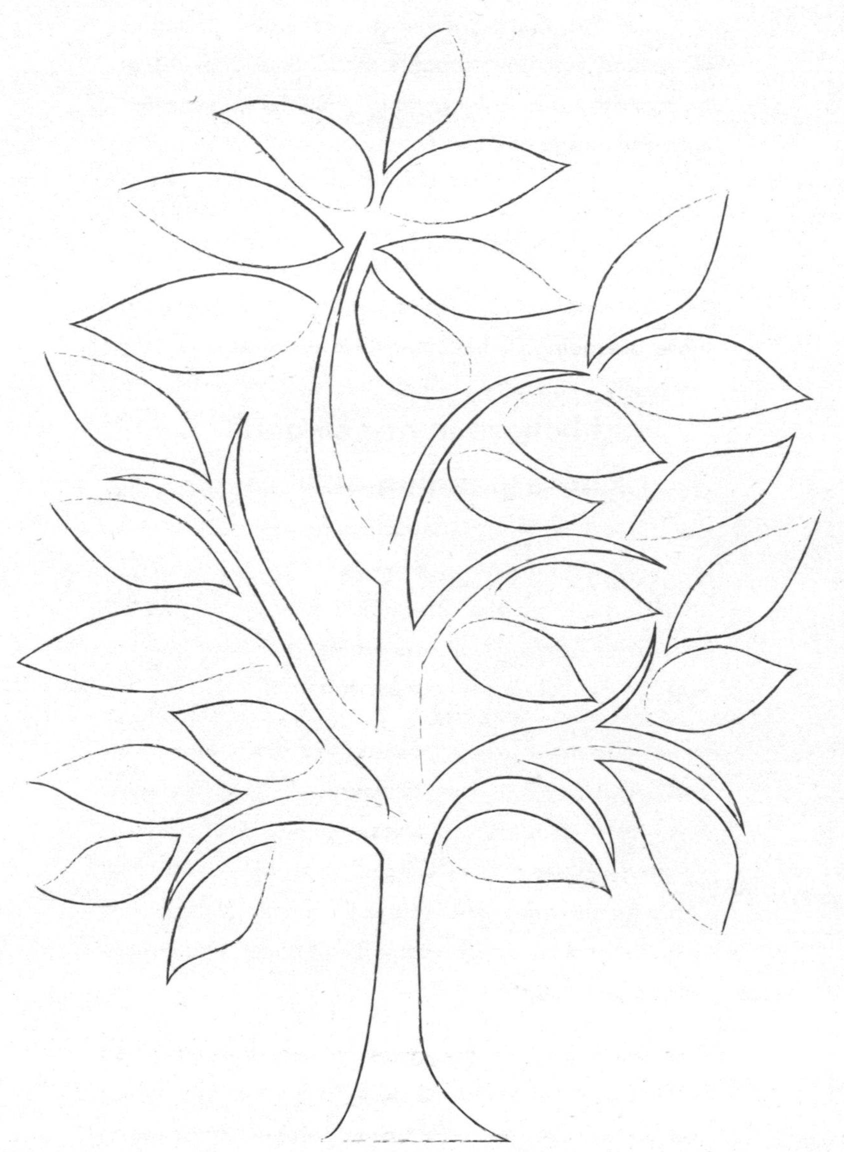

self-belief. Drawing on these strengths and strategies will remind you how capable and adept you are at dealing with difficult things, and you'll feel a renewed sense of courage and clarity in no time.

I believe in myself and my expanding abilities

A FINAL THOUGHT

As your baby continues to grow into childhood and beyond, so do you. You are learning together and you are navigating new adventures and challenges all the time. Please make space to acknowledge how far you have come, and do this regularly. The upside-down/inside-out nature of motherhood often makes our progress hard to quantify, but with every smile your baby gives you, know that you are doing truly incredible work.

Continue to speak kindly to yourself, cut yourself some slack and prioritise regular rest and replenishment. Reward yourself with time and softness. Motherhood is the most demanding job there is and the more you look after yourself, the more you have to lovingly give.

Remember that you are still you. You are you, expanded. You are you with more compassion, more love, more vulnerability, more courage and a wider range of skills than you ever realised. And this is still just the beginning. As your child continues to grow you will remain their beacon of love and safety. Never, ever underestimate the value of this work. You are changing the world.

ACKNOWLEDGEMENTS

When I finished writing my first book, I could never have envisaged writing another one, so my first expression of gratitude goes to Sam Jackson, my commissioning editor, for convincing me to do it again. Your belief in me and your support for me is so appreciated. Thank you to my brilliant editors – Leah Feltham and Jacqui Lewis — for the time and expertise you've given to *Motherhood Your Way*, and to the whole team at Ebury who are among the most professional I've ever been lucky enough to work with. A huge thank you to Emma Scott-Child and the team at Junction Studio for bringing this book to life with your perfect illustrations. Thank you to my literary agent, Jessica Stone at Independent, and to the Tape Agency team who have welcomed me so warmly into their family.

My heartfelt thanks to all of the people I've been lucky enough to teach and work with, in all of your glorious forms. It is always a privilege and I learn so much from you. This book wouldn't exist without your everyday experiences and your willingness to share, learn and grow with me. A huge thank you to everyone who has bought, shared, supported and read this book, too. How lucky I am to write for such a wonderful bunch of people!

Thanks to Jill Thompson – the best therapist I've ever known. You have taught me so much about myself and my place in the world, and it's really changed my life for the better.

Thank you to the friends who've put up with me being missing in action for the most part of this writing process. Your understanding and compassion means so much to me: Amanda Frost, Charlotte Crook, Clemmie Telford, Jo Stainton, Kate Hughes, Liz Matthews, Roxanne Houshmand-Howell, Jane Scotting, Sarah Macadam, Sophie Ardern, Susan Foynes, Steve Ball, Tayo Popoola, Vanessa Hurley. You are all absolute gems.

To the friends who continue to make my motherhood experience with Cosmo such an absolute joy: Becks Clarke, Caroline Collins, Frankie Farnesi, Kat Bee, Lorna Hayward – I cannot tell you how grateful I am for each one of you. You are not only incredible mothers, but some of the most caring, generous and devilishly funny women I've ever been lucky enough to meet.

Thank you to the women who inspire me professionally every day, but especially when I think of what's gone into this book: Annie Francis, Beccy Hands, Carly Hardman, Illiyin Morrison, Imogen Unger, Izzy Judd, Laura Brand, Nancy Nunn, Rene Bozier, Tekie Quaye.

Warmest of thanks to our wonderful nanny, Lydia, for loving Cosmo as much as you do and being such a loving and valuable part of our family. I couldn't have written this book without knowing my baby was in such safe and capable arms.

To the people I've missed most in this strange year – my wonderful family. Thank you to my amazing parents for your unwavering support over the last 36 years and for understanding that I never answer my phone. Thanks to my brother Jack and his wife Laura for being incredible in many ways this year, and of course to Archie, too. Thank you to Keith and Irene for making my parents happy and loving them like you clearly do. Thanks and love to Heike and Anthony for the love and support you show to me and the boys, and to Simon's family who have welcomed me so warmly. We are lucky to have you all. And to my grandparents, Mama and Gandy – without knowing, you set me up on the path to writing this book. You always encouraged me to be myself and loved me so wholly for it. Gandy, it's very hard to navigate this life without you in it any more, but thank you for showing up when you do. I see and feel you so often and I love it.

Thank you a million times over to Simon, the absolute love of my life. Your faith in me and love for me is something I feel so grateful for every day. You've brought more to my life than you'll ever know, and I couldn't feel happier to be navigating the ups and downs of all of our adventures with you. You are such an incredibly loving dad and our boys are so very lucky. Having you and Manolo in my life will forever be a blessing.

Lastly, to Oscar and Cosmo. What a privilege it is to be your mother. Oscar, your softness, strength and unparalleled kindness is an absolute joy to watch. Never stop standing up for yourself and for fairness. It is a rare and beautiful gift and something I am so proud of you for. Cosmo, thank you for the light you brought back to my life. The magic you see in the simplest of things really inspires me, and your cheeky, knowing, sparkly-eyed spirit is just divine. You will both have my love and encouragement always. Wherever you go, whatever you want to do, whatever challenges you encounter along the way – I'm right behind you and always will be.

And to the mothers. You have more of an impact on this world than anyone else. Your love is what we need. It is always the remedy, it is always the answer.

INDEX

Page references in *italics* indicate images.

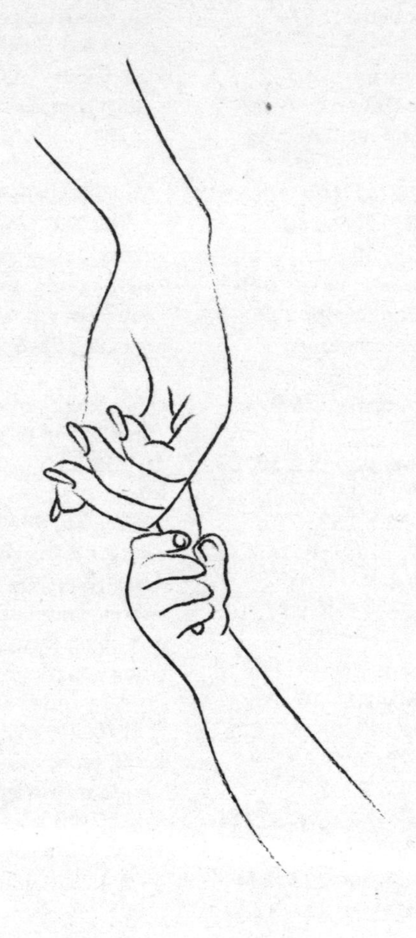